A Manual for Acute Postoperative Pain Management

A Manual for Acute Postoperative Pain Management

Ferne B. Sevarino, M.D.
Associate Director, Acute Pain Services
Department of Anesthesiology
Yale University School of Medicine
New Haven, Connecticut

Linda M. Preble, R.N., M.P.S.
Clinical Administrator,
Pain Management Services
Department of Anesthesiology
Yale University School of Medicine
New Haven, Connecticut

with contributions by

Jim G. Weeks
Vice President, Business Development
Medical Management Incorporated
Montgomery, Alabama

Raymond S. Sinatra, M.D., Ph.D.
Director, Acute Pain Service
Department of Anesthesiology
Yale University School of Medicine
New Haven, Connecticut

RAVEN PRESS 🦢 NEW YORK

Raven Press, Ltd., 1185 Avenue of the Americas, New York, New York 10036

Made in the United States of America

Library of Congress Cataloging-in-Publication Data

Sevarino, Ferne B.
  A manual for acute postoperative pain management / Ferne B.
Sevarino and Linda M. Preble.
     p.   cm.
  Includes bibliographical references and index.
  ISBN 0-88167-866-X
  1. Pain, Postoperative—Treatment. 2. Pain clinics. I. Preble,
Linda. II. Title.
  [DNLM: 1. Outpatient Clinics, Hospital—organization &
administration. 2. Pain, Postoperative—therapy. 3. Postoperative
Care.   WL 27 S497m]
  RB127.S43   1992
  362.1'960472—dc20
  DNLM/DLC
  for Library of Congress   91-32850
                                                                        CIP

The material contained in this volume was submitted as previously unpublished material, except in the instances in which credit has been given to the source from which some of the illustrative material was derived.

Great care has been taken to maintain the accuracy of the information contained in the volume. However, neither Raven Press nor the editors can be held responsible for errors or for any consequences arising from the use of the information contained herein.

9 8 7 6 5 4 3 2 1

Contents

Preface

The inadequacy of postoperative pain management is commonly discussed in medical literature (1–6). Despite increased attention toward this issue, the majority of patients treated with parenteral opioids continue to experience inadequate analgesia (1). A lack of understanding on the part of the medical community regarding optimal methods of treatment and the significant morbidity associated with undermedication, has led to the development of dedicated specialists and pain management services.

This manual provides guidelines for establishing and maintaining an Acute Pain Service, which offers hospitals a team of clinical specialists best suited to manage acute pain. The basics of formulating analgesic therapy are outlined in Chapters 1–5. Patient management is discussed in Chapters 6–12. Key references have been included that outline the more important aspects of acute pain management, including organization, policy and procedures, drug delivery, and treatment of adverse events.

The protocols and recommendations presented in this book were developed during the first three years of operation of Yale University/Yale–New Haven Hospital Acute Pain Service. Although such protocols work well at our institution, we recognize that other departments face different hospital policies and may have different goals and needs. Drugs, dosages, mode of administration, and indications are our recommendations and may not be FDA approved for these purposes. We hope that much of the material presented will, nevertheless, aid in the development of Acute Pain Services at other institutions.

Ferne B. Sevarino
Linda M. Preble

REFERENCES

1. Cronin M, Redfern PA. Psychometry and postoperative complaints of pain in surgical patients. *Br J Anaesthiol* 1973;45:879.
2. Marks RM, Sachar EJ. Undertreatment of medical inpatients with narcotic analgesics. *Ann Intern Med* 1973;78:173–181.

3. Loper KA, Butler S, Nessly M, Wild L. Paralyzed with pain: the need for education. *Pain* 1989;37:315–316.
4. McCaffrey M, Beebe A. *Pain: clinical manual for nursing practice.* St. Louis: CV Mosby Co., 1989.
5. Perry SW. The undermedication for pain. *Psychiatr Ann* 1984;14:808–809.
6. Schuchman M, Wilkes MS. Suffering in silence. *New York Times* July 23, 1989.

SUGGESTED READING

Cancer pain relief. Geneva, World Health Organization, 1986.
Jong R H. Defining pain terms. *JAMA* 1980;244:143.
Merskey II. Pain terms: a list with definitions and notes on usage, IASP subcommittee on taxonomy *Pain* 1979;6:249–252.

Acknowledgments

We would like to thank Dr. Paul Barash for his encouragement and support, and Marie Warner for her humor and secretarial skills.

A Manual for Acute Postoperative Pain Management

PART I

The key to a successful Acute Pain Service is detailed planning and organization, with a systematic approach to implementation and expansion. In this section of the manual, we have presented a step-by-step approach to the essential aspects of this process.

1

Traditional Postoperative Pain Management

Pain is among the most common symptoms encountered in the hospitalized patient (1). It is a subjective experience (2), the perception of which varies from individual to individual. The International Association for the Study of Pain (IASP) defines pain as the sensory and emotional experience associated with actual or potential tissue damage or described in terms of such damage (9).

Although newer methods of controlling pain are available and, if properly applied, can relieve or even prevent suffering, the analgesic technique still most commonly prescribed by physicians is intramuscular injection of opioids administered every 3–4 hr on an "as needed" basis. Dosage has traditionally been determined on a standardized, nonindividualized basis with little or no evaluation of its effectiveness (3). A number of variables—including patient age, physical status, extent of surgery, and the individual patient's coping skills—affect the adequacy of pain relief (4). Traditional therapy, unfortunately, does not address these variables. This often leads to ineffective treatment with inadequate dosage and/or inappropriate intervals between doses of medication (5). The result is a recurring cycle of pain, gradual relief, excessive sedation, and the return of pain (1) (Fig. 1.1). Evaluations of "on demand" dosing schedules have revealed that analgesic plasma concentrations of opioid are attained for less than one-third of the treatment cycle (5) (Fig. 1.2).

The undertreatment of pain may be further magnified by the nursing staff (2). Traditional pain medication orders include a drug, dose, and an interval range. The nurse often chooses the smallest dose from the prescribed range and/or chooses the longest interval between dose administration. The effectiveness of pain treatment may further be hindered by patients themselves, who often will not request or take the prescribed medication, fearing addiction or other complications. Thus, undermedication arises from a lack of understanding of opioid pharmacokinetics/pharmacodynamics by health

3

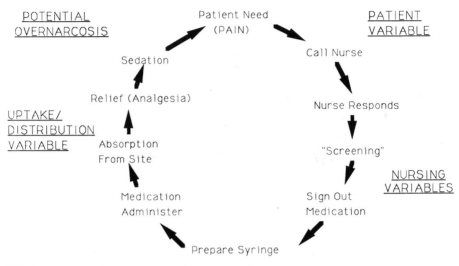

FIG. 1.1. Delay between the perception of pain and effective relief with conventional analgesic therapy.

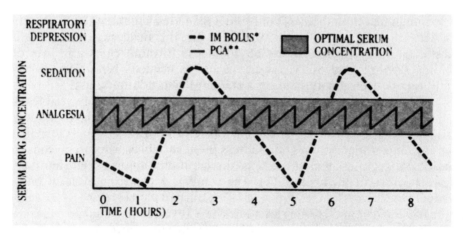

FIG. 1.2. IM dose-response compared to PCA dose-response objective. Reprinted with permission from Abbott Laboratories.

care providers, the fear of overdosing the patient on the part of the prescribing physician and the nurse administering the analgesic, and the concerns of the patient himself (2).

Pain that is undertreated can lead to physiologic complications, including respiratory compromise and an increased cardiac workload (6) (Fig. 1.3). The patient may also suffer psychological distress, manifested by demoralization, social withdrawal, behavioral regression, temper tantrums, and belligerent behavior. Both the physiologic and psychologic consequences of undertreated pain affect—either directly or indirectly—the patient and all others involved. The patient's distress affects his/her family, and frustrates both the nurse and physician; the treatment of pain *must* be considered a priority and ideally individualized for each patient (2). To individualize therapy, one must rely on the patient to indicate the degree of his/her pain. The patient must be provided with an assessment scale, most often a verbal pain scale (2) or visual analogue scale to quantify the intensity of their pain (see Chapter 6). Such measurement will serve as a basis for evaluating pain intensity and for assessing the adequacy of subsequent therapy. There must also be a mechanism for altering pain management regimens to allow individualization of therapies. An individual who understands the interactions of opioids and who has a broad knowledge of modalities for pain management must be central to this process (7).

Uniquely qualified to treat acute postoperative pain is the anesthesiologist. Training and knowledge of opioid, nonopioid, and local anesthetic pharmacology, as well as the understanding of pain pathways and mechanisms, and the experience with regional anesthesia, are necessary to optimize the management of acute pain (8). Anesthesiologists have long

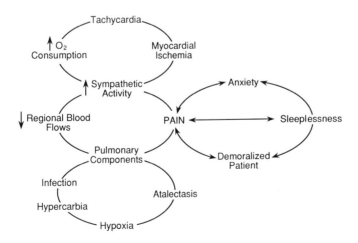

FIG. 1.3. Harmful effects of unrelieved acute pain.

recognized that there are more similarities than differences among the numerous opioid derivatives, and in order to achieve greater efficacy of pain management, more appropriate methods of drug administration are required. New pain management techniques include, among others, patient-controlled intravenous analgesia, spinal opioid analgesia, interpleural analgesia, and continuous plexus analgesia. To best accommodate the anesthesiologist's expanding role outside the operating room, many Departments of Anesthesiology have formed Acute Pain Management Teams, and thus have established Acute Pain Management Services.

REFERENCES

1. Cronin M, Redfern PA. Psychometry and postoperative complaints of pain in surgical patients. *Br J Anaesthiol* 1973;45:879.
2. McCaffrey M, Beebe A. *Pain: clinical manual for nursing practice.* St. Louis: The CV Mosby Co., 1989.
3. Marks RM, Sachar EJ. Undertreatment of medical inpatients with narcotic analgesics. *Ann Intern Med* 1973;78:173–181.
4. Gravis D, Foster A, Batenhorst RL. Patient controlled analgesia. *Ann Intern Med* 1983;99:360–366.
5. White PW. Management of post-operative pain use of opioid analgesics. *IARS Review Course Lectures* 1987;84–89.
6. Brown DL, Carpenter RL. Perioperative analgesia: a review of risks and benefits. *J Cardiothoracic Anesthiol* 1990;4:368–83.
7. Hull CJ. Pharmacokinetics of opioid analgesia, PCA. In: Harmer M, Rosen M, eds. *Patient controlled analgesia.* Oxford: Blackwell, 1985.
8. Ready LB. Rational choice of postoperative analgesic techniques. *Anesthesiol Rep* 1990; 2:194–199.
9. International Association for the Study of Pain. Core Curriculum for Professional Education in Pain. IASP Publications, Seattle, 1989.

SUGGESTED READING

Donovan M, Dillon P, McGuire L. Incidence and characteristics of pain in a sample of neurosurgical inpatients. *Pain* 1987;30:69–78.
Ready LB, Oden R, Chadwick HS, et al. Development of an anesthesiology-based postoperative pain management service. *Anesthesiology* 1988;68:100–106.
Sriwatanakul K, Weis OF, Alloza JL, et al. Analysis of narcotic analgesic usage in the treatment of postoperative pain. *JAMA* 1983;250:926–929.
Ulting JE, Smith JM. Postoperative analgesia. *Anaesthesia* 1979;34:320–332.

2

Anesthesiology Based
Acute Pain Service

As stated in Chapter 1, the anesthesiologist is uniquely qualified to direct the Acute Pain Service (APS). Organizationally, the Pain Management Service must be a functionally dedicated team without operating room responsibility (1–3).

A team of dedicated individuals must be available to provide patient care, which includes daily rounds, consultations, 24-hr housestaff coverage, etc. A consultative APS team allows for the standardization and safe delivery of analgesic therapy. Newer techniques require the education of both health care providers and patients to their use, and the APS provides the mechanism for this education. The team is a discrete service that integrates into the organization of the healthcare facility, yet maintains the separate identity it needs and deserves. The availability of trained personnel helps to ensure safe delivery of analgesic therapy provided by patient-controlled analgesia (PCA), intrathecal and epidural opioids, interpleural analgesia, or other modalities. The Clinical Director of the APS works with the Clinical Nurse Coordinator to develop orders, treatment protocols, and policy to ensure maximum efficacy and patient safety.

The goals of the Acute Pain Team in any setting are (a) to provide optimal analgesia; (b) to individualize pain management therapy; and (c) to be responsive to the patient's needs (2). The team assists the operating room anesthesiologists in the planning of the postoperative analgesic care for their patients and provides consultation to the surgeon for postoperative pain management. Also important is the formal and informal education provided to healthcare providers. In an academic setting, the APS also provides training and education for resident physicians who will carry this knowledge into their own practices. The academic based pain service also has a mandate to undertake research utilizing new agents and techniques with the ultimate goals of improving patient care, improving analgesia, and decreasing morbidity.

7

To ensure success, the APS must function as a 24-hr, 7-day/week consultative service (1–5). A member of the APS is available at all times to handle referrals of patients undergoing emergency surgery and to provide an immediate response to medical emergencies (4–6). The manner in which this coverage is provided, as well as the exact role of the APS, will be influenced by the type of practice setting (community versus academic) (Table 2.1). In a community practice, an anesthesiologist and/or Certified Registered Nurse Anesthetist (CRNA) provides this coverage. In academic practices, coverage is usually provided by resident physicians who are available in hospital and who have attending physicians available for "back-up." In either setting, all team members should possess a fundamental understanding of the pain management techniques used and be able to interact effectively with the hospital community. Table 2.2 outlines goals and objectives for individual team members. Table 2.3 outlines guidelines for an APS (7).

TABLE 2.1. *Unique aspects of academic and community practices*

Type of practice	Characteristics
Academic practice	To provide leadership for the development of effective services.
	To clarify in a scientific manner, the most effective/optimal forms of treatment and their safe applications.
	To train future anesthesiologists in the management of acute postoperative pain.
	Recommended number of attending anesthesiologists is between 4 and 8, with one responsible attending at any one time.
	Rotation schedule is a *must* (ie., daily, weekly, monthly rotations).
	No other clinical responsibilities when assigned to the APS. (In some institutions, the APS attending also provides patient care in the Chronic Pain Center.)
	Fellow/resident availability to provide 24 hr in-hospital coverage.
Community practice	To meet the needs of their patients efficiently and effectively.
	To standardize the service.
	To provide extensive nursing education.
	To provide 24 hr coverage of the service problems/emergency surgery:
	In a setting with no in-house, 24-hr coverage by an anesthesiologist or CRNA, the anesthesiologist covering the APS must be willing to make prompt hospital visits when necessary.
	In a practice where night coverage is available by an in-house anesthesiologist and/or CRNA, their support may be utilized for night coverage of patients on the APS.
	Possibly hiring CRNA's or Registered Nurses to provide 24-hr, in-house coverage. The anesthesiologist must be available by beeper in the event of an emergency.
	A minimum of 2 anesthesiologists alternate night/weekend coverage.

TABLE 2.2. *Pain service team members: Goals and objectives of the individual members of the APS*

To understand pain and its mechanisms
  Pharmacokinetics and pharmacodynamics of opiates
  Pain pathways

To be knowledgeable about pain assessment
  Distinguish pain from anxiety
  Ability to assess pain
  Evaluation of effectiveness of traditional pain therapy versus new pain management
    therapies

To be knowledgeable about PCA
  Understand the rationale for PCA—physiology/pharmacology
  Utilization of equipment
  Medications available for PCA and the dose ranges for effective therapy
  Side effects and their treatment
  Appropriate responses to therapy; the ability to distinguish between inadequate dosing and
    overdosing

To be knowledgeable about spinal (epidural/intrathecal) opioids
  Understand the rationale—physiologic/anatomic
  Medications available: dose ranges
  Postoperative care of epidural/intrathecal catheters
  Treatment of side effects
  Pharmacologic principles of epidural/intrathecal solutions

To be familiar with alternative therapies, including
  Interpleural analgesia
  Intercostal blocks
  Stellate ganglion blocks
  Lumbar sympathetic blocks
  Cervical plexus blocks
  Caudal blocks
  Ankle blocks
  Oral narcotics and nonnarcotic analgesics

To be visible within the hospital community
  Develop interpersonal and communication skills
  Develop relationship with other healthcare providers
  Instruct nursing personnel, patients, and surgical staff as to availability, risks, and benefits
    of various pain therapies

TABLE 2.3. *Guidelines for an APS*

Careful patient selection, adjusting opioid doses for patient age and physical status
Routine follow-up
Education of all nursing personnel regarding the use and risks of all pain management
  modalities
Regular nursing education updates
Use of printed protocols and standard orders developed jointly by physicians and nurses to
  govern the use of the new pain management modalities
Continuing quality assurance

Adapted from ref. 7.

REFERENCES

1. Hammonds WD, Reed B, Kelly P, Sands P. Pain management team. *Anesthesiol Rep* 1990;2:148–154.
2. Ready LB, Oden R, Chadwick HS, Benedetti C, Rooke GA, Caplan R, Wild LM. Development of an anesthesiology-based postoperative pain management service. *Anesthiology* 1988;68:100–106.
3. Ferrell BR, Wenzl C, Wisdom C. Evolution and evaluation of a pain management team. *Oncology Nursing Forum* 1988;15:285–289.
4. Carr DB, McPeek B, Todd DP, Ryder E. So you want to start a postoperative pain service? *J Clin Anesthesiol* 1989;1:320–321.
5. Ready LB, Wild LM. Organization of an acute pain service: training and manpower. *Anesthesiol Clin North Am* 1989;7:229–239.
6. Benzon HT. Postoperative pain and its management. *Resident and Staff Physician* 1989;35:21–26.
7. Gwirtz KH. Intraspinal narcotics in the management of postoperative pain. *Anesthesiol Rev* 1990;17:16–28.

3

ABC's of Starting a Pain Service

PLANNING

Personnel

To ensure the overall success of the APS, the commitment of key personnel is essential to the planning, organization, and implementation of the service (Fig. 3.1).

Director

The Clinical Director, an anesthesiologist, should be responsible for the startup initiative and maintenance of the Acute Pain Service (APS). The

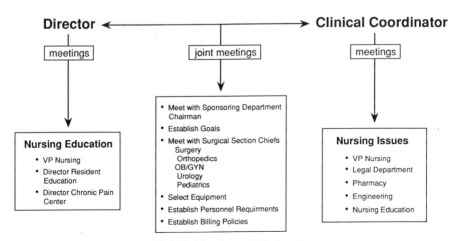

FIG. 3.1. Planning a Pain Service.

11

commitment of this individual to the program and its progress is key to its effectiveness (1,2). The director should ideally have fellowship training in pain management or extensive knowledge of pain management techniques and opioid pharmacology. The responsibilities of the Clinical Director are to (1) hire and supervise the Clinical Nurse Coordinator (CNC); (b) in conjunction with the CNC, establish orders and policy for pain management; (c) interact with the hospital administration; (d) do public relations/education; (e) act as the contact person for surgeons, hospital personnel, and patients for this part of the Department of Anesthesiology's practice; (f) recruit interested Attending Anesthesiologists to participate in the service; and (g) do resident education and evaluation (Fig. 3.1).

Clinical Nurse Coordinator

The CNC (see Table 3.1 for job description) is responsible for the day-to-day functioning of the APS. (S)he reports regularly to the director. (S)he is the individual who interacts on a regular basis with patients, nurses, consulting physicians, pharmacists, and administrators, and thus provides the greatest continuity of care (3). (S)he is the most visible individual on the service. The Clinical Director usually has other responsibilities, including operating room responsibilities and other clinical and on-call duties; thus, the CNC is dedicated to overseeing the day-to-day operation of the service, and reporting to the director.

Ideally, the CNC should be a Registered Nurse with experience on the patient care floors and postanesthesia care unit (PACU). (S)he must be experienced in interacting with nursing staff, supervisors, and administrators. A CRNA is unlikely to have extensive experience outside the operating room and is therefore less suited for this role than a Registered Nurse, who has the experience mentioned above.

The responsibilities of the CNC are tailored to the type of institution (academic or community) and may include (a) clinical and/or administrative duties; (b) consultative assistance; (c) research and academic publication; (d) education of healthcare personnel and patients; (e) establishment and evaluation of nursing standards of care regarding pain management; (f) establishment of quality assurance guidelines; and (g) develop both formal and informal education programs for nursing personnel (Fig. 3.1).

Other Personnel

In addition to the director and CNC, additional physician and nursing staff are necessary for the day to day operations of the APS (1–3). See Table 3.2 for the staffing of the APS at Yale–New Haven Hospital/Yale University School of Medicine (Fig. 3.1).

TABLE 3.1. *Yale–New Haven Hospital: Job Description for Clinical Coordinator, APS, Department of Anesthesiology*

Summary
  Reports to the Director of the APS and is responsible for the following: Establishment and evaluation of standards of care in the Acute Pain Management area; planning and implementation of educational programs for Nurses, Surgical and Anesthesiology Residents; coordination of patient care, education and monitoring of participants; organization of patient data collections. (S)he serves as a consultant and resource person to all members of the patient care team.

Position duties and responsibilities
  Participates in the establishment, implementation and evaluation of standards of care for patients in the APS and serves as a consultant in the inpatient setting to health professionals and patients.
  Collaborates with the Pharmacy Department to provide the appropriate medication for each patient and return charging procedures.
  Serves as a consultant to the company representatives for equipment necessary to APS function.
  Evaluates the Pain Service, both formally and informally, to improve and ensure the quality of its care and programs, and implements into standards of care appropriate research findings.
  Assesses consultation requests of referring physicians and assists the APS physician in determining suitable pain treatment regimen and its application.
  Performs a variety of duties, both clinical and administrative, to support the smooth operation of the APS.
  Plans, implements and presents pain management programs for nursing, surgical and anesthesia personnel.
  Interviews prospective candidates for postoperative pain treatment, educates and explains the nature of the program. Educates nursing staff and patients on PCA pumps.
  Identifies and systematically investigates clinical and clinically related problems and communicates these results to Pain Service Care Team for discussion.
  Performs other job related functions when necessary.

Position specification
  Position title: Clinical Coordinator, APS
  Position reports to: Director, APS, or Vice President of Nursing or designated appointee, if hired by Department of Nursing
  Education (that amount of formal education normally required to perform the position duties): RN and Master's Degree with a concentration in Management/Administration
  Experience (number of years and type required to meet an acceptable level of performance): Minimum two (2) years experience involving clinical administrative and research project management and program coordination.
  Special skills: Excellent interpersonal, clinical and organizational skills. Background in Obstetrics/Gynecology or postanesthesia care preferred.
  Coordinates all administrative, patient care, and research activities of the APS. Ensures appropriate monitoring, communication with and follow-up of participating patients throughout the program. Coordinates and ensures necessary data collection and reporting.
  Complexity (describes planning, problem solving, decision making, creative activity or other special factors inherent in the responsibilities of this position): Determines appropriateness of patient participation in the program. Provides education to patients and appropriate hospital personnel. Strong interaction with Pharmacy and PCA company representative.

TABLE 3.2. *APS at Yale–New Haven Hospital: Staffing*

Personnel	Duties
Director	See Chapter 3
Attendings (13)	Provide APS coverage on a weekly basis. Coverage of the service is easiest from Monday through Sunday, with no additional clinical responsibilities Monday through Friday. Faculty, however may be assigned in-house call on Saturday or Sunday. Attend/give morning lectures. Make rounds on all patients with the Clinical Nurse Coordinator, resident and fellow. Round with resident on weekends. Determine type and duration of therapy for patients. See all consults and counter-sign all follow-up notes. Participate in clinical research.
Fellow (1)	Responsible for one or more monthly lectures. Make rounds. Participates in clinical studies. Assists the attending/resident in patient management and consults. On back-up call to the resident.
Residents (3)	Assigned to APS for 1 month. One resident provides 24-hr APS coverage (in-house), one resident is off (post-call), and the clinical responsibilities of the third resident are in the Chronic Pain Center.
Clinical Nurse Coordinator (1)	See Chapter 3
Assistant Clinical Coordinators (2)	Primarily responsible for clinical care. Working hours are as needed for clinical duties: one nurse available for morning rounds, and one in-house until 8 or 9 pm to assist the resident as needed. Ensure adequacy of equipment and supplies. Provide nursing inservices. Ensure that billing forms are completed and sent to billing department. Assist the resident as needed in initial assessment of the patient for enrollment in the Pain Service. Assist in clinical research. At Yale–New Haven Hospital, the Clinical Nurse Coordinator and assistants ensure that standards of care are clearly communicated to the nursing staff; physician orders are clear and concise; and the responsibilities of staff nurses are understood. They act as a liaison between APS physicians and other healthcare providers.
Pharmacist	In some institutions, the pharmacist dispenses the analgesics and infusions as ordered by the APS and has no further role. Yale–New Haven Hospital is working towards making the pharmacist a member of the team, who will make recommendations, provide information and thus become more directly involved in patient management.

There is a single beeper number for the APS. This beeper is carried by the APS resident covering for the day. All hospital personnel use this beeper number for consultations or problems.

Site Visits

Following the appointment of a director and the hiring of a CNC, the next step should be for both individuals to visit other institutions with established APS's. Ideally, the service visited should be similar in scope to the one being planned, i.e., community-based versus academic-based service, large or small institution.

Suggested Agenda for a Site Visit

Day one:
Spend the morning with the APS
   a. Attend lecture and morning report
   b. Accompany the team on morning patient rounds
Review the following topics with the appropriate personnel:
   a. Director: Pain management therapies (e.g., drugs, doses, methods), medical management of patients, surgeons' acceptance of the APS within the administration's acceptance of the service.
   b. CNC: Policies and procedures, charting and narcotic distribution, order sheets, consult sheets, billing sheets, teaching materials/articles, and inservice protocols (see Appendices 1.1–1.9).
   c. Business Manager: Coding and billing procedures, equipment, and supplies.
Day two:
Leave unscheduled to allow for further discussion, questions and observations (Fig. 3.1).

Intrahospital Planning Meetings

Following the site visit, the director and CNC should meet with the appropriate personnel in their own hospital (Table 3.3, Fig. 3.1).

ORGANIZATION

Organization of the APS is a process that will require approximately 3–4 months to complete (Fig. 3.2). During this phase, the important aspects of the APS are addressed: standardization of orders (Appendix 1.8), charting (Appendix 1.7), and the delineation of responsibilities (Appendix 1.2). This is the most critical phase and should be undertaken carefully to ensure quality patient care and maximize the efficiency of the APS. Table 3.4 outlines the organizational process.

TABLE 3.3. *Planning the APS*

APS Personnel	Hospital/Dept. Personnel	Agenda
Director and CNC	Chairman, Department of Anesthesiology	To establish goals, personnel requirements, and time frame for implementation of the service.
	Department of Anesthesiology Business Manager	To develop budget and discuss billing options.
	Board of Trustees	To present the concept and anticipated role of the Pain Service.
	Surgical Sections Chiefs	To present the concept and role of APS as a consultative service.
	Vice-President of Nursing	To discuss nursing involvement and support.
	Company Representatives	To examine equipment and supplies.
	Hospital Finance Committee	To discuss the impact of the new service on hospital budget.
Director	Director of Resident Education (in academic practice)	To determine resident manpower requirements, for departments with residency training programs.
		To determine goals and objectives of the pain service rotation for the residents.
CNC	Policies and Procedures Committee Chairperson	To design and write nursing policies and procedures.
	Director, Pharmacy	To discuss and determine: Narcotic disbursement and charting Handling narcotic proof-of-use sheets Standard allotments and drug appropriation Disbursement—individual patient vs. storage in patient care units. Arrange purchase of new narcotic doses, if necessary Prefilled syringes vs. pharmacy prepared syringes Drug incompatibilities
	Director, Engineering Department	To establish service procedure—repairs, safety checks, maintenance, technical requirements.
	Director, Medical Records Department	To discuss charting requirements, use of pretyped order forms, and preprinted follow-up notes.

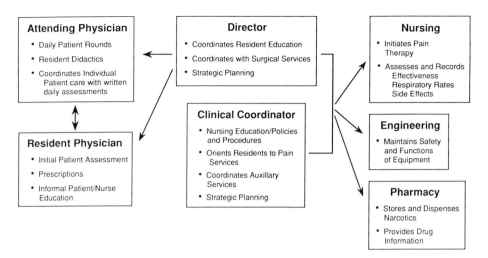

FIG. 3.2. Organizing an Acute Pain Service.

IMPLEMENTATION

Upon implementation, predetermined educational curricula and plans for expansion should be followed (Fig. 3.3).

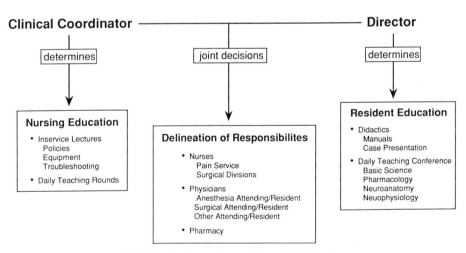

FIG. 3.3. Implementing an Acute Pain Service.

Education

A formal education program will provide the means for a systematic introduction of the APS and its role in pain management.

TABLE 3.4. *Organization of the APS*

	Agenda
Strategic planning	Define the type (PCA, epidural, and/or other) and location (floor, ICU, etc.) of services to be provided.
	Prepare a business plan to clarify objectives.
	Estimate patient volume targets.
	Study the insurance mix at the institution.
	Determine reasonable charges for the services provided.
	Determine which equipment will be used.
	Determine who (department vs institution) will own/lease equipment, and who will charge for supplies.
	Determine manpower needs (see Table 3.2).
Financial planning	Determine initial financial outlay.
	Determine salary expenses.
	Determine nonsalary expenses.
Logistics	Develop the necessary forms (i.e., consult sheets, data sheets, follow-up notes, billing forms).
	Develop standard orders and design order forms.
	Equipment and supplies:
	Central supply location vs storage on patient care units
	Distribution of equipment
	Cleaning and maintenance of equipment
	Determine where pain management will be initiated and by whom.
	Post Anesthesia Care Unit vs patient care unit
	Nursing personnel vs Pain Service personnel
	Delineate responsibilities
	Pharmacy
	APS
	Nursing Care Units
	Biomedical engineering safety inspection of equipment
	Determine who will be responsible for analgesic orders when pain management therapy (PCA, epidural, interpleural, etc.) is discontinued: The primary physician or the APS physician.

Nursing Education

The support of the Department of Nursing is necessary for the success of the service (3). Every nurse must participate in formal, structured inservice programs prior to the institution of any new pain management techniques on any particular patient care unit. Appendix 1.1 outlines patient-controlled analgesia (PCA) and epidural inservice programs. Programs for interpleural analgesia, caudal analgesia, and nerve blocks follow the same format. The primary focus of any nursing inservice is on nursing diagnosis and responsibilities. Regularly scheduled updates should also be provided. The staff nurse, as the healthcare provider with the greatest degree of patient interaction, must be able to assess pain, evaluate the effectiveness of pain management, and be able to identify the side effects and drug interactions (Appendix 1.9) that occur. The APS team relies on the input of the staff nurse for safe and effective patient care. During the implementation phase, the CNC and her/his assistant are the primary resource people for nursing personnel. They must be available continually, as this will greatly alleviate the apprehension and uncertainty of the nursing staff upon initiation of the new program. The quality of patient care is strengthened by the maintenance of a good working relationship with the nursing staff. Nursing standards are established early in the planning and organizational stages; they are utilized in the implementation stage. The governing documents are the policies and procedures, which outline standards of care within the institution. Guidelines, although not binding, are the "working documents." They are more detailed in nature and provide the bedside nurse with examples of assessment and charting and include, for example, drug incompatibilities and other relevant information. Appendix 1.2 contains policies and procedures from several institutions; Appendix 1.3 contains nursing guidelines. These should be adapted to meet the needs of the individual institution and the Nursing Practice Act of each state.

As pain management becomes technologically advanced, many hospitals require their nurses to attend a formal inservice, which includes a practical and written examination and thus allows for credentialling (see Appendix 1.4). Nurses must show proficiency before (s)he provides care for patients whose pain management includes newer techniques (PCA, epidural analgesia, interpleural analgesia, etc.). The choice of inservice procedures for the APS is joint, made by the CNC, nursing education, and nursing administration.

Physician Education

Anesthesiology Staff

The Attending Anesthesiologist is provided with a list of physician responsibilities. Staff meetings are scheduled on a regular basis to discuss problems, new pain management therapies, and other information relevant to the APS. Departmental grand rounds should be conducted by the Clinical Director of the APS approximately every 6 months to update the department on changes within the service. Resident education should be undertaken (see Appendix 1.5).

Nonanesthesiology Physician Staff (Surgeons, Pediatricians, Hematologists, Oncologists, Other House Staff, Etc.)

Formal education, which is usually provided at the individual departments' grand rounds, should cover the following: (a) The APS is a consultative service for pain management; it is stressed that the pain service does not provide or interfere with the surgical or medical management of patients. Although the patient is under the care of the APS, the surgeon (resident or attending) will be contacted by the nursing staff for any problem not related to pain management. (b) Pain management options and the benefits/risks of each modality are discussed. (c) Responsibilities of the APS are outlined; if PCA or neuraxial narcotics are employed, the APS is responsible for all pain therapy and sedative orders.

Patient Education

Patients should be made aware of the options available to them for postoperative pain management. Many vendors provide patient education pamphlets which may be included in the prehospital admission packet or given to the patient in the primary physician's office or upon admission to the hospital (see Appendix 1.6). Ideally, information should be provided prior to admission to the hospital.

Marketing an APS

Consider advertizing in the hospital newsletter and through the newspaper and/or telephone book. Be available for interviews with the lay press. Emphasize the benefits to the patient of this service as provided by your hospital (see Chapter 5).

Expansion of the Pain Service

Expansion should proceed in a logical, progressive manner, expanding/growing either patient care unit by patient care unit or by surgical service. It is essential that a smooth transition be made from traditional pain management modalities to the newer techniques. Staff nurses must be educated on pain assessment, be kept up-to-date about new drugs available for pain relief, and inserviced on the new equipment utilized for pain management. One should not attempt to provide acute pain management care for the entire institution at the onset. Expanding step-by-step allows for an organized formal approach to the introduction of all aspects of the newer modalities. Without nursing acceptance and support, the service will not succeed.

Summary

The establishment and maintenance of an APS requires administrative commitment, including a close liaison with the nursing staff to develop appropriate educational and procedural standards. Interaction with surgeons, house staff, hospital pharmacists, and those providing the surgical anesthesia care is essential. For the service to be well-planned and organized, its personnel must be dedicated, and possess considerable forethought, organization, planning, and commitment (1,2,4). Table 3.5 presents the daily operations of the Acute Pain Service at Yale–New Haven Hospital/Yale University School of Medicine. (Figures 4–8 are further clarification found in this table.) This system works well in our institution and, with modification, should work in other institutions.

TABLE 3.5. *The APS at Yale–New Haven Hospital/Yale University School of Medicine: Operation*

Daily schedule
  Morning lecture at 7:30

  Sign out rounds
    Following the morning lecture, the resident going off duty reports on the status of each patient, including diagnosis, therapy and problems that have occurred during the previous 24 hr.

  Morning rounds
    Depending on the number of patients on the service, one or two teams may round. As Monday typically is our lightest day, only one team makes rounds. When there are 30 or more patients to be seen in the morning, the team is split. Patients are divided equally between the two teams, which consist of one nurse and one physician. Both teams see patients from each of the surgical services: i.e., gynecology, obstetrics, orthopedics, urology, general surgery, and pediatrics, as each group of patients presents different problems. The team sees every patient and assesses the quality of analgesia (VAS pain and satisfaction scores), the presence or absence of side effects and whether or not these side effects have been adequately treated. If necessary, therapy is adjusted. A progress note, *signed by the attending anesthesiologist,* and a continuation/discontinuation order is written for each patient (Fig. 3.4). Following rounds, the team reconvenes and reviews all of the patients. Pain management therapy is reevaluated for any patient with whom there has been a problem. ICU patients and consultations are seen by the attending, resident and fellow. For the remainder of the day, the resident is available to see consultations, to enroll new patients into the Pain Service, and to manage problems.

  Enrollment of patients
    A patient is enrolled with the APS after consultation with and approval by, the patient's surgeon. A written postoperative consultation request must be made. The analgesic orders are written in the PACU and an initial consultation form is completed. In the PACU, the consultation form is completed by a physician member of the APS and analgesic orders are completed.

    The initial consultation forms at YNHH consist of three pages: the top sheet includes pertinent medical information and the plan of therapy, and is placed in the patient's history and progress notes (Fig. 3.5). The second and third pages are utilized by the APS: the second is an individual data sheet, filled out daily and kept in a nursing log book, and the third is the billing sheet.

  Physician log book
    The resident carries a log book containing a record of each patient on the service with pertinent medical information, currently administered medications, allergies, and pain therapy (Fig. 3.6).

  Nursing log book
    A loose leaf book containing a data sheet and billing sheet (Figs. 3.7 and 3.8) on each patient is kept up to date daily. Data is used for assessing adequacy of individual treatment as well as the efficacy of a treatment for the patients as a group.

  Afternoon rounds
    Afternoon rounds are made by the attending, resident, fellow, and clinical nurse coordinator or assistant. Patients seen at this time include new patients, all ICU and pediatric patients, and all those with problems that were noted on morning rounds.

  Evening rounds
    The resident is encouraged to round again in the evening. We find that this facilitates communication with both patient and the nursing staff and greatly reduces the number of phone calls made to the resident in the middle of the night.

The patient is currently on day _____ of management by the Pain Service

Therapy: PCA _____, Epidural _____, Other _____

        Drug and dose _____.

Response Scale (0-10): Pain _____; Satisfaction _____.

Side Effects: None _____, Nausea/vomiting _____, Itching _____,
             Drowsiness _____, Respiratory depression _____
             Confusion _____.

Treatment: _____.

Assessment of epidural catheter site: _____.

PLAN: Therapy to continue _____; Therapy to be discontinued today _____;

      Therapy to be changed as follows:_____

_____

_____.

Date: _____   _____ M.D.

FIG. 3.4. Department of Anesthesiology—Pain Service. Follow-up notes.

YALE UNIVERSITY SCHOOL OF MEDICINE
DEPARTMENT OF ANESTHESIOLOGY
PAIN SERVICE CONSULT

LOCATION	PRIMARY PHYSICIAN/REFERRING SURGEON	ATTENDING ANESTHESIOLOGIST		

ANESTHESIA NURSE OR RESIDENT	YR AGE MO	ASA STATUS	SURGICAL SVC	SEX

DATE OF INITIAL SERVICE	DIAGNOSIS/PROCEDURE	PAIN LOCATION

PLAN:

The patient will receive: PCA   Epidural   Other

Drug and dosage   _____

_____

The patient has been referred for optimization of analgesia and will be followed by the Pain Service twenty-four (24) hours a day while on the service.

Pertinent Clinical Information: _____

_____

_____

_____

_____

_____

Medications _____

Allergies _____

Instructions:

The patient has received instructions and educational information and is aware of potential risks regarding PCA/epidural narcotics.

Other _____

Residents, attendings, and nurses have been instructed on patient care and that no additional narcotics or sedatives should be administered while the patient is followed by the Pain Service.

The nursing staff has been given explicit orders for the care of the patient and guiodelines when to call the Pain Service.

Date _____   _____ M.D.

FIG. 3.5. Yale University School of Medicine Department of Anesthesiology Pain Service Consult Form. Part A.

```
NAME _____

AGE_____  ROOM #_____

  PROCEDURE _____

RX  _____

    _____

    _____

START                          STOP
DATE _____  TIME _____  DATE_____
      1     2     3     4     5     6

HX  _____

    _____

MEDS  _____

  KDA  _____
```

FIG. 3.6. Example of a page from a Physician Log Book.

LOCATION	PRIMARY PHYSICIAN/REFERRING SURGEON		ATTENDING ANESTHESIOLOGIST	

ANESTHESIA NURSE OR RESIDENT	YR AGE MO	ASA STATUS	SURGICAL SVC	SEX

DATE OF INITIAL SERVICE	DIAGNOSIS/PROCEDURE	PAIN LOCATION

CONSULT LEVEL						
DATE						
DAY	1	2	3	4	5	6
PRIM AGENT						
PRIM TECH						
2ND AGENT						
2ND TECH						
SUPPLEMENTAL MEDS						
24 HR TOTAL						
SIDE EFFECTS/Rx						
VAS REST MOVEMENT						
VAS SAT						

SIDE EFFECTS VAS SCORES

N/V = 10   0-10
Pruritus = 11
Urinary Ret = 12
Resp. Depression = 13
Confusion = 14
Sedation = 15
Dizziness = 16

AGENTS

Meperidine - 16	Duramorph - 38
Morphine - 17	Narcan - 39
Fentanyl - 18	Reglan - 40
Other Narcotics - 20	TD Scop - 41
Bupivacaine - 22	Dilaudid - 42
Lidocaine - 24	Midazolam - 43
Diazepam - 2 6	Sufentanil - 44
Droperidol - 27	Benadryl - 45
	Phenergan - 46

TECHNIQUES

Thoracic Epidural - 41
PCA - 42
Cont via PCA pump - 43
PCA + CONT - 44
Intrapleural Blk - 45
Brach Plex Infus - 46
Nerve Block (para vertebral) - 71
Lum Sympathetic - 78
Intercos Nerv Blk - 81
Peridural: lum - 84
Peridural: lum cont - 85
Spinal - 87
Other moethods - 91

FIG. 3.7. Yale University School of Medicine Department of Anesthesiology Pain Service Consult Form. Part B.

YALE UNIVERSITY SCHOOL OF MEDICINE
DEPARTMENMT OF ANESTHESIOLOGY
PAIN SERVICE CONSULT

LOCATION	PRIMARY PHYSICIAN/REFERRING SURGEON		ATTENDING ANESTHESIOLOGIST	
ANESTHESIA NURSE OR RESIDENT	YR AGE MO	ASA STATUS	SURGICAL SVC	SEX
DATE OF INITIAL SERVICE	DIAGNOSIS/PROCEDURE		PAIN LOCATION	

CONSULT LEVEL						
DATE						
DAY	1	2	3	4	5	6
CPT CODE						
FEE						

TOTAL

LEVELS OF CARE:

Limited: 90250-75 (PCA Day 3)
Intermediate: 90260-75
Extensive: 90270-75 (PCA Day 2)
Comprehensive: 90280-75

DIAGNOSIS:

Pain of:

_____ Head - 7840	_____ Face, Atypical - 3502	_____ Arm - 7295
_____ Neck - 7231	_____ Hip - 71945	_____ Ankle - 71947
_____ Back - 7245	_____ Groin - 7890	_____ Knee - 71946
_____ LBP - 7242	_____ Shoulder - 71941	_____ Neuralgia - 7292
_____ Face - 7840	_____ Neuroma - 2159	_____ Other ( )

FIG. 3.8. Yale University School of Medicine Department of Anesthesiology Pain Service Consult Form. Part C.

REFERENCES

1. Ready LB, Oden R, Chadwick HS, Benedetti C, Rooke GA, Caplan R, Wild LM. Development of an anesthesiology-based postoperative pain management service. *Anesthesiology* 1988;68:100–106.
2. Ready LB, Wild LM. Organization of an acute pain service: training and manpower. *Anesthesiol Clin North Am* 1989;7:229–239.
3. Hammonds WD, Reed B, Kelly P, Sands P. Pain management team. *Anesthesiol Rep* 1990; 2:148–154.
4. Ferrell BR, Wenzl C, Wisdom C. Evolution and evaluation of a pain management team. *Oncology Nursing Forum* 1988;15:285–289.

SUGGESTED READING

Hord A H, Kokenes C. Postoperative pain: a review of management methods. *Hosp Formul* 1989;24:28–38.

4

Billing and Coding Strategies and Alternatives for Acute Pain Management

Jim G. Weeks

To better understand some of the issues surrounding the billing and coding of professional services for acute pain management, we need to examine the history of this service.

With the demand for better and more dedicated pain care, and the advances in technology, drugs, and treatments, there has arisen a need for specialized medical and management attention to this issue. The anesthesiologist, for reasons discussed in earlier chapters, has been placed in the forefront of this rapidly growing service. Unfortunately, the rapid growth of this consultative service did not allow for advance planning or consultation with most third party payers or public agencies. In addition, certain therapies have been sporadically offered without the help of specialists, and the resulting confusion has created uncertainty in the reimbursement positions of payers.

Although there was greater understanding among payers regarding the role of the anesthesiologist for epidural case management, this knowledge was not universal and there remain regional pockets of confusion. Intravenous therapies [e.g., intravenous patient-controlled analgesia (IV-PCA)] presented the provider with a new set of problems. There were no specific codes with which to clearly identify the service rendered. This led to significant experimentation on the part of providers, inconsistent or improper documentation of services, and confusion among providers and payers.

The following will address some of the current issues surrounding the billing and payment of acute pain management professional services. We will also discuss important points of consideration when dealing with payers, as well as the long-term payment prospect.

THIRD-PARTY PAYER PERSPECTIVE

Why Pain Management?

A lack of understanding here can prevent any further discussion with payers. Appropriate clinical documentation should be presented.

Why Anesthesiology?

Don't we pay the surgeon for this already? Why can't the nurse handle it? Don't we pay anesthesiologists to provide postoperative care? These are some typical responses of payers, indicating a genuine lack of knowledge regarding acute pain therapies, as well as the need to individualize therapy, and the importance of providing consistent medical supervision. Additionally, the carriers and providers are unfamiliar with anesthesiology services provided outside of the operating room.

LEVEL OF PAYER AWARENESS

No Specific Notice

This position is typically seen when services are not providing care for a significant number of patients. It is inadvisable to believe this position would be long-lasting. One must develop a plan to deal with the issues as they come up.

Investigation of Coverage/Payment

If this is the case, it is imperative to educate the payer community by providing documentation which shows the critical role of the anesthesiologist in assuring safe and effective treatment for the patient.

Inadequate Payment Levels and Inappropriate Coverage Guidelines

Once a carrier/payer has established less than adequate payment levels for the service or severely restrictive coverage guidelines, it becomes far more difficult to negotiate to a reasonable position. It is imperative that the reeducation process be well considered and organized. At this point, it may be necessary to seek outside counsel and assistance from local or state societies. This is not a totally negative situation, since there is usually some acknowledgment of the appropriate therapist's role in the course of treatment.

CODING FOR ACUTE PAIN MANAGEMENT
PROFESSIONAL SERVICES

One might surmise that the type and level of service provided would dictate the coding for professional services. Unfortunately, this approach does not always work for pain management services. In fact, dependent upon local payer issues we see a variety of acceptable coding options. As a general rule, the epidural coding is simpler than other pain management modalities or therapies as it typically is a surgical service with identifiable procedure codes. The choice of coding options will be influenced by practice specific realities or specific payer preferences.

Table 4.1 denotes codes that are primarily used when billing for epidural catheter insertion and usually include associated services provided by the physician on the first postoperative day. Less frequently, they are repeated for subsequent daily management. It is generally considered inappropriate to charge separately for this procedure if the catheter is used to administer anesthesia during the surgical procedure and there is a specific charge for the anesthesia. Some carriers have specified that no additional payment will be made.

Codes for intravenous therapy especially those for initial consultation, were used by the early acute pain services and remain the dominant coding channel in several regional service areas (Table 4.2). The most frequently seen codes are 90600, 90610, and 90620. The follow-up consultation or confirmatory consultation are rarely used. When the initial consultation option is used in addition to the appropriate service(s) outlined in the Current Procedural Terminology (CPT–90), it usually includes the first day of service postoperatively or with a medical patient the first full day of service.

TABLE 4.1. *Epidural coding options*

Code	Procedure
62274	Injection of anesthetic substance (including narcotics), diagnostic or therapeutic; subarachnoid or subdural, single
62276	Subarachnoid or subdural, differential
62277	Subarachnoid or subdural, continuous
62278	Lumbar or caudal epidural, single
62279	Lumbar or caudal epidural, continuous
62288	Injection of substance other than anesthetic, contrast, or neurolytic solutions; subarachnoid (separate procedure)
62289	Lumbar or caudal epidural
63780	Insertion, subarachnoid or epidural catheter, with reservoir and/or pump for drug infusion, without laminectomy
01196[a]	Daily management of epidural or subarachnoid drug administration

[a]This code is currently the predominant code for subsequent daily care of the pain management patient with an indwelling epidural catheter. The use of this code is not restricted by use of the catheter for anesthesia. In such circumstances, this code is used on each postoperative day.

TABLE 4.2. *Intravenous coding options: Consultations*

Code	Type of consultation
Initial consultation	
90600	Initial consultation; limited
90605	Intermediate
90610	Extended
90620	Comprehensive
90630	Complex
Follow-up consultation	
90640	Follow-up consultation; brief
90641	Limited
90642	Intermediate
90643	Complex
Confirmatory (additional opinion) consultation	
90650	Confirmatory consultation; limited
90651	Intermediate
90652	Extended
90653	Comprehensive
90654	Complex

FOR REVIEW WHEN ESTABLISHING BILLING PRACTICES

Provider Numbers

History would support the use of a separate provider number for pain management services to avoid confusion with traditional anesthesia and to facilitate tracking of revenues from each business sector. In some areas, it may be difficult to obtain additional provider numbers.

Claim Terminology and Detail

When completing the claim form, attention to detail is paramount. A complete and correct description of the service provided, along with appropriate type of service code, diagnostic code, and referring physician when needed are essential. Incorrect terminology or inappropriate type of service and diagnostic coding are the most common problems with denied claims.

Participation, Assignment, and Patient Billing Options

It is important to evaluate these options carefully when establishing your service. Your current participation contracts may refer only to traditional services thus allowing you to go outside those contracts for new services such as pain management. When considering your patient billing options, it might be helpful to contact other providers of similar services in your area or seek outside counsel as to the optimal/accepted billing practices in your area.

ELEMENTS OF SUCCESS IN "PLANNING AND PREPARATION"

Physician Commitment

The support of your partners and surgical and medical colleagues will be essential to the success of the program. This support must be earned and reinforced on a continuous basis.

TABLE 4.3. *Hospital medical services (new and established patient) billing codes*

Code	Type of care
Initial hospital care	
90200	Initial hospital care; brief history and examination, initiation of diagnostic and treatment programs, and preparation of hospital records
90215	Intermediate history and examination, initiation of diagnostic and treatment programs, and preparation of hospital records
90220	Comprehensive history and examination, initiation of diagnostic and treatment programs, and preparation of hospital records
Subsequent hospital care[a]	
90240	Subsequent hospital care, each day; brief services
90250	Limited services
90260	Intermediate services
90270	Extended services
90280	Comprehensive services
Infusion therapy	
90280	IV infusion therapy, administered by physician or under direct supervision of physician; up to 1 hr
90781	Each additional hour, up to 8 hr. This coding channel is infrequently seen and its use is quite localized.
Therapeutic or diagnostic injections	
90784	Intravenous. This option is rarely seen and is typically payer specific.
Other options	
01999	Unlisted anesthesia procedure(s). This particular code usually represents infrequently provided services or procedures such as intrapleural infusions. It is usually accompanied by an extensive operative report when the claim is filed.

[a]To date, the most frequently used codes have been 90240 and 90260 in conjunction with the initial consultation codes. There is significant variance between regional service areas.

Financial Plan

An in-depth financial plan outlining all identifiable costs for the practice or department and the hospital should be prepared prior to service initiation. A *reasonable* revenue projection for the practice and the hospital is critical.

Goal Development and Strategic Planning

Reasonable goals should be set and agreed upon by all parties. A monitoring process should be established to check the progress of the business plan. A plan should be developed which includes a strategy to educate specific payers when necessary. Here again, outside consultation with experts and other providers would be helpful.

Summary

The recommendations in Tables 4.1–4.3 are suggested ways of coding for pain management services. It may be more expeditious to contact other service providers in your area and seek outside counsel prior to establishing your service.

LONG-TERM PAYMENT PROSPECTS

Achievement of the following goals will help assure the success of the service:

Medically necessary therapies and services
Reasonable charges reflecting service provided
Superior service on a consistent basis
Proper and consistent documentation and coding
Community value must be established

Although much work is yet to be done, significant progress has been made toward developing appropriate coverage guidelines and reasonable payment levels.

The progress of the service will be aided by the coordination of efforts with local, state, and national societies, and the determination of those individuals driving such efforts.

5

Marketing an Acute
Pain Service

Marketing is targeted communication that requires effective listening and response to the needs of the group to be served (1). It is an often used technique in industry and is now being used in the healthcare sector. The marketing of services offered by an institution can promote the hospital's image and bring additional financial resources into the hospital (2).

Direct marketing of an Acute Pain Service (APS) is difficult because the service is provided upon referral by a primary physician (surgeon, internist, pediatrician) and, thus, volume is dependent upon the referral base. To gain support, the APS should formally discuss its role within the hospital and discuss new pain management modalities that are available for patient care. This is best done at surgical/medical grand rounds. Further, the director and Clinical Nurse Coordinator (CNC), should be readily accessible to the primary physician to provide informal inservices and address concerns. If the primary physician has a positive attitude toward the service, that attitude translates into referrals.

The patient must also be made aware of the service, and must be satisfied that the service is providing care that is in his/her best interest. Patients will communicate their level of satisfaction or dissatisfaction to their friends and family (3). This will affect prospective patients, who will be inclined either to request referral to the service or not. Patient information packets regarding the pain service should be included in the admission information sent to patients. (See Appendix 1.6.) The APS at Yale University/Yale–New Haven Hospital has a patient questionnaire that is mailed to patients several weeks after discharge from the hospital. Figure 5.1 outlines this survey. We also provide the patients with a card listing the names of individuals involved with the service (Fig. 5.2). All comments/criticisms of the service are answered personally by the director/associate director or Clinical Nurse Coordinator.

Dear   :

     As Director of the Acute Pain Service, Department of Anesthesiology, it is helpful for me to know your impressions of the care you received from the Pain Service while you were a patient at Yale-New Haven Hospital. Would you please take a minute to complete the following questions and return this sheet in the envelope provided?

                      Sincerely,

                      Director,
                      Acute Pain Service

1.   Did the Center for Pain Management personnel demonstrate genuine concern?

        Unsatisfactory   1 2 3 4 5 6 7 8 9 10   Satisfactory

2.   Were you given an adequate opportunity to discuss your concerns, likes, dislikes regarding your pain management therapy?

        Unsatisfactory   1 2 3 4 5 6 7 8 9 10   Satisfactory

3.   Overall, how would you rate the care you receivied from the Center for Pain Management?

        Unsatisfactory   1 2 3 4 5 6 7 8 9 10   Satisfactory

4.   Any additional comments: _____

_____

_____

_____

_____

FIG. 5.1. APS Yale–New Haven Hospital Patient Survey.

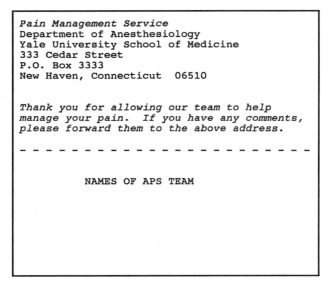

FIG. 5.2. APS Public Relations Card.

Advertising is usually the mode of marketing with which most people identify (1). Healthcare organizations often publish an in-house newsletter to promote the institution, its staff, and services. Articles about the pain service published in this in-house paper keep the staff aware of new services available (Fig. 5.3). Indirect marketing can be achieved through newspaper exposure.

To summarize, a referral service such as the APS must be advertised to those physicians who are the referral base and sold to the patient, without whom there is no service (Fig. 5.4).

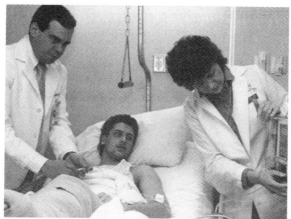

Patient Travis Knotts watches closely *as Linda Preble, clinical coordinator of the new Acute Pain Service, and Dr. Raymond Sinatra, director of the program, check his PCA—patient-controlled analgesia.*

New Pain Service Brings Relief to Many; Patients Control Own Analgesia Delivery

It didn't look good for 19-year old Travis Knotts. At the printing company where he works, a 2,000-pound roll of paper fell and crushed his left leg. He was rushed to Yale-New Haven Hospital and operated on. Fortunately, three orthopaedic reconstructive surgeries saved his leg.

Though it hasn't been easy for Travis, one thing he doesn't complain about is the pain.

"The pain hasn't been too bad," Travis said from his hospital bed on the eve of his third operation.

The reason? Travis, like an increasing number of YNHH patients, is using patient-controlled analgesia (PCA), which has enabled him to administer his own pain medication.

What makes it possible for patients to receive PCA in lieu of single injections of pain medications, is the department of anesthesiology's newly created Acute Pain Service (APS). The service is on call 24 hours a day to prescribe pain medications, provide follow-through care and closely monitor each patient.

"Patients are constantly staying ahead of the pain with PCA; it never becomes overwhelming," notes Raymond S. Sinatra, M.D., Ph.D.,

assistant professor of anesthesiology at the School of Medicine and director of the APS. "It doesn't make the pain go away entirely, but it brings it down to a very tolerable level on a consistent basis," he adds.

Research Leads to New Service

The Acute Pain Service was established after three years of research by medical center physicians. Since the new, sophisticated PCA methods require continual monitoring, physicians realized that an organized effort was needed to bring their research to the bedside. Close supervision, back-up service and education to nurses were needed.

The pain service also offers nerve block injections and continuous epidural pain relief (using a catheter inserted in the spinal column through which pain medications are fed). Gynecological, obstetrical, intensive care and orthopaedic patients benefit from the program. Eventually, the service will reach the entire hospital.

In addition to Dr. Sinatra, the service is staffed by clinical coordinator Linda Preble, R.N., M.S.N., attending physicians and anesthesia residents.

PCA, which is heralded as a revolutionary and exciting pain relief method, not only controls pain quickly, but also frees up nurses' time and allows patients to get out of bed sooner. It is administered via a computerized infusion pump containing a syringe filled with the medication. The pump is directly attached to the patient's I.V. pole. A control panel feeds information into the machine on the type of medication being used, maximum allowed dosage and minimum intervals between doses. By squeezing a hand-held device similar to a nurse-calling button, the patient triggers the system, which is usually attached through a vein in the hand.

YALE NEW-HAVEN MEDICAL CENTER **LIFE**

A newsletter published five times a year for the faculty, students and staff of Yale-New Haven Hospital, Yale School of Medicine and Yale School of Nursing.

Co-editors: Gregory Huth
Katie Krauss

Contributors: Sharon Bass, Mary Colwell, Leah D'Eugenio, Helaine Patterson, Bruce Reynolds and Paula Runlett.

The deadline for the Summer issue of MEDICAL CENTER LIFE is April 15.

FIG. 5.3. Newsletter Information about the APS.

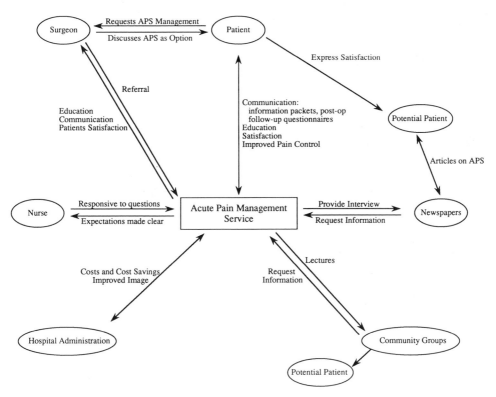

FIG. 5.4. Referral Networking.

REFERENCES

1. Goldsmith SM. *Health care management. A contemporary perspective.* Rockville, IL: Aspen Systems Corp., 1981.
2. Welnetz K. Marketing a continuing education course for healthcare managers. *Journal of Continuing Education in Nursing* 1990;21:62–67.
3. Johnson J. Clarkson rewrites the book on hospital marketing. *Hospitals* 1990;November 20:33–34.

Appendix 1.1: Nursing Education

PCA INSERVICE

Session I is a lecture. This lecture includes:

A. Introduction to the pain service
    1. Organization
    2. Structure
    3. Function
        a. PCA
        b. Spinal opioids (with emphasis on epidurally administered opioids)
        c. Consultations
B. Definition of PCA
    1. History
    2. Explanation of optimal analgesia
    3. Advantages of optimal analgesia
    4. Safety factors
C. Responsibilities
    1. Acute pain service physician
        a. Initial patient assessment—introduce consult forms
        b. PCA prescription—introduce standard orders. Discussed during this phase are:
            1. Drug choices for PCA
            2. The pharmacodynamics and pharmacokinetics of the more commonly prescribed medications
            3. Usual dosage and dosing intervals
            4. The importance of protocol for administering additional opioids/sedatives
            5. Possible side effects and available treatments
            6. Assessment responsibilities
            7. Guidelines for immediate notification of the APS
    2. Nursing: This portion focuses on the initiation of therapy, with an emphasis on setting up the pump and the signing out and recording of opioids used, assessing and recording the effectiveness of therapy, monitoring (frequency of vital signs, pulse oximetry) to assure patient safety and charting responsibilities (respiratory rates, level of analgesia, level of sedation, side effects, and treatment).
D. Trouble shooting of equipment
E. Drug incompatibilities (see Appendix 1.9)

    Session II is a hands on clinic, and is mandatory for each staff nurse. It emphasizes learning to program the PCA pump per the written prescription, making appropriate changes in therapy when ordered, and handling and recording opioids used.

SPINAL OPIOID INSERVICE

A. Introduction to the APS
    1. Organization
    2. Structure
    3. Function
        a. Consultations
        b. Spinal opioids
        c. PCA
B. Epidural analgesia
    1. Anatomy
        a. Pain pathways, opioid receptors
        b. Catheter placement and opioid administration—difference between epidural and intrathecal opioid administration
    2. Drugs utilized
        a. Different opioids and their uses
        b. Usual doses
        c. Sites of administration (lumbar vs. thoracic)
        d. Intermittent injection vs. continuous infusions
        e. Concomitant use of local anesthetics
    3. Side effects and treatment
C. Responsibilities
    1. APS physician
        a. Initial pain assessment—introduce consult forms
        b. Prescription—standard orders are introduced and the importance of a protocol for administering parenteral opioids/sedatives is discussed. Patient assessment and guidelines for immediate notification of the APS is emphasized.
        c. Patient assessment—frequency of physician assessment of the patient is discussed, VAS pain scores are introduced, and follow-up notes are reviewed.
    2. Nursing
        a. Assessment and documentation of the effectiveness of therapy
        b. Charting: respiratory status, level of analgesia, level of sedation, side effects and treatment, and condition of catheter insertion site.
        c. Appropriate handling and recording of opioid usage

Based upon the Nursing Practice Act of the respective state, each institution will determine who is to be responsible for the administration of intermittent boluses and/or the initiation and maintenance of continuous infusions. If nursing personnel are to be responsible, it will be necessary to develop further formal inservicing clinics for proficiency in injection techniques and criteria for gaining credentials.

INTERPLEURAL INSERVICE

A. Interpleural analgesia
   1. Explanation of optimal analgesia
   2. Indications for use of interpleural analgesia
   3. Anatomy and physiology
      a. Anatomy of chest wall
      b. Insertion techniques
      c. Positioning of patient
   4. Complications
   5. Use of local anesthetics
      a. Intermittent injection vs. continuous infusions
      b. Usual dosages
      c. Signs of toxicity
      d. Incidence of toxicity
   6. Breakthrough pain
      a. Positioning the patient
      b. Treatment options
         1. Opioids
         2. Opioid agonist-antagonists
         3. NSAIDs
B. Responsibilities
   1. APS
      a. Insertion of catheter
      b. Initial patient assessment—introduce consult forms
      c. Prescription—standard orders are introduced
   2. Nursing
      a. Continued assessment of the patient
         1. effectiveness of therapy
         2. respiratory status
         3. monitoring of vital signs
         4. catheter insertion site
         5. monitoring for signs and symptoms of local anesthetic toxicity

Within each institution and within the scope of each state's Nursing Practice Act, nursing must address their role and responsibilities to administer intermittent interpleural injections, and/or initiation and maintenance of continuous infusions.

Appendix 1.2: Policies and Procedures

POLICIES AND PROCEDURES
(GOVERNING DOCUMENT)

Policies and procedures are standards of care and are followed by the entire nursing staff. They are approved by the Vice President for Nursing, the Chief of Staff, the Chairman of the Department of Anesthesiology, the Director of the Department of Epidemiology Infection Control, and the Director of Pharmacy Services. The following policies and procedures have been adapted from those used at Yale–New Haven Hospital and may be further adapted to conform to individual institutional constraints.

PATIENT CONTROLLED ANALGESIA: POLICY I

I. General statement of purpose

This policy and procedure is for nursing professionals who will be caring for patients using an IV PCA infusion device for the delivery of controlled substances prescribed for acute (postoperative) and chronic (intractable) pain management by the APS—Department of Anesthesiology.

The purpose of this method of administering pain medication is to give the patient a sense of control over his/her pain and provide a more effective dosing method for the administration of a controlled substance.

II. Definition

PCA allows for the intravenous administration of small amounts of opioid at frequent intervals, keeping blood levels of the opioid within an effective range. Excessive or inadequate levels of opioid in the blood are thereby avoided, and periods of either excessive sedation or ineffective pain control are reduced.

III. Guidelines

A. SYSTEMIC CONTROLLED SUBSTANCES OR SEDATIVES SHALL NOT BE GIVEN WITHOUT NOTIFYING THE ACUTE PAIN SERVICE. UNLESS SPECIFICALLY STATED, PATIENTS MAY RECEIVE MEDICATION FOR SLEEP WHILE ON PCA (except patients receiving a basal infusion—they may not have sleeping medications unless the APS resident is notified).

B. Patients who would not normally receive parenteral opioids, and those either physically or emotionally incapable of using the PCA device, are not suitable candidates for PCA therapy.

    C.   PCA therapy may be deemed appropriate for certain individuals under the age of 5 or 6.

    D.   Naloxone, 1 ampule (Narcan 0.4 mg/ml), should be available in the patient's unit dose cassette in the event that it becomes necessary to reverse the effects of the PCA opioid.

    E.   PCA therapy is administered intravenously by a PCA infusion device that is locked at all times. Two keys are kept for the infusion device, one with the controlled substance cabinet keys on the patient care unit, and the other with the APS Resident.

    F.   A malfunctioning PCA infusion device is replaced as needed.

    G.   Nonsterile, disposable gloves are to be worn when manipulating or changing the intravenous catheter device.

    H.   Controlled substances for PCA are supplied in syringes and stored in the locked controlled substance cabinet. They are audited as schedule II controlled substances.

    I.   All nursing personnel, before providing care to patients using a PCA infusion device (this includes the initiation or changing of PCA parameters, and changing the PCA substance syringe), are required to attend inservice classes, given by the Department of Anesthesiology/Nursing Education Department.

IV. Responsibilities

    A.   APS Physician, Department of Anesthesiology

        1.   Explains the risks/benefits and potential complications of PCA therapy

        2.   Writes prescriptions for each patient which include:

            a.   Controlled substance, milligram/cc, basal rate, PCA increment, delay time, and 4-hr limit

            b.   Availability of naloxone hydrochloride

            c.   Antiemetics to be administered

            d.   Frequency of respiratory assessment

            e.   Discontinuation of all prescriptions for controlled substances and other central nervous depressants while the patient is on PCA

        3.   If he/she initiates PCA, records required information on the controlled substance proof of use sheet

        4.   Administers naloxone hydrochloride as required, and provides appropriate documentation

    B.   Registered Nurse

        1.   Verifies the presence of a complete written prescription for PCA on the "Doctor's Order Sheet"

        2.   Maintains a patent intravenous catheter

        3.   Has knowledge of the following:

       a. Risks/complications and benefits of intravenously administered opioids

       b. Pharmacology of drug administered

       c. Immediate and long-term side effects of intravenously administered opioids and appropriate interventions when necessary

4. Has current Basic Life Support certification
5. Knows how to contact the APS Resident physician
6. Confirms the presence of naloxone hydrochloride in the patient's unit dose cassette
7. Initiates PCA, changes pump syringes, and changes PCA dose as ordered after completing inservice classes
8. Records the necessary information on the controlled substance Proof of Use Sheet when initiating, changing or terminating a PCA pump syringe
9. Discards, with a witness, any controlled substance not utilized, and documents this on the Proof of Use Sheet
10. Monitors the patient and documents the patient's response to therapy
11. Documents any nursing interventions taken
11. Notifies the APS resident physician if the patient:

       a. Has respiratory rate of less than 10 breaths/min

       b. Is somnolent or confused

       c. Complains of pruritus

       d. Has urinary retention

12. Consults, when necessary, with the APS Clinical Nurse Coordinator.

V. Monitoring

  A. Checks the respiratory rate as prescribed by the anesthesiologist, and records this information on the Daily Patient Care Record

  B. Assesses and documents the following in the history and progress notes every 4 hr for the first 24 hr and then every shift thereafter while on PCA:

     1. Level of analgesia

     2. Level of consciousness

  C. Assesses the patient with respect to the following every shift:

     1. Nausea and vomiting; if present, treat as ordered

     2. Pruritus

     3. Urinary retention

  D. Records the amount of medication (in milligrams) administered by the patient through PCA device every eight hours on the "Medication Administration Record" (MAR)

PATIENT CONTROLLED ANALGESIA: POLICY II

The PCA Infuser is an instrument designed to permit patient controlled delivery of parenteral analgesic drugs. Medications, dosage to be given and time intervals are prescribed by the physician. Patient Monitor: Registered Nurse.

Policy

Patient Selection

A. Eligible patients
   1. Patients requiring parenteral analgesic medications
      a. Postoperative pain relief
      b. Chronic pain syndromes
      c. Trauma patients
   2. Mentally alert patients. Patients must be able to understand and follow instructions and be physically capable of operating the PCA infuser
   3. Patients *without* a history of allergy to the prescribed opioid
B. Ineligible Patients
   1. Confused patients that limit their ability to self-administered medication
   2. Pregnant or nursing women unless opioid analgesia is clearly indicated

The suitability of candidates for the use of the PCA infuser will be made by the attending physician of the patient or his designee.

Patient Information

Patient instruction will be provided to all who utilize the device. Each patient should receive clear instructions on the PCA infuser prior to having the device set up. These instructions will be given by the nurse caring for the patient. When the PCA infuser is to control postoperative pain, the instructions should be given on the day prior to surgery. Prepared instructions will be given to the patient and explained. The patient and the instructor will sign the sheet when the teaching is completed. The completed sheet should be sent to the pharmacy.

Physician Prescribing Analgesia per PCA Infuser:

The physicians order *must* contain the following: (a) name and strength of drug; (b) loading dose volume (ml); (c) incremental dose volume (ml); (d) lockout interval (min); and (e) 1° hour volume limit (ml).

Loading Dose

This can be given if the patient has pain before the use of the PCA infuser has begun.

Incremental or PCA Dose Volume

This is the amount administered each time the patient activates the PCA infuser.

Lockout Interval

This is the period of time that must pass between the completion of one dose and the initiation of the next. The PCA infuser cannot be activated and no medication is delivered. This allows time for the dose to take effect and the patient is able to assess relief before asking for another dose.

One-Hour Volume Limit

This is the maximum volume that will be delivered by the PCA in one hour.

Pharmacy Protocols

1. The dispensing of the cartridge will be on a written physicians order only.
2. Nursing units will requisition cartridge on controlled substance floor stock requisition. Patient name and room number must be included on requisition.
3. Vials will be dispensed with a controlled substance administration record. One vial per administration record.
5. A running log of shift usage will be kept and signed by the nurse caring for the patient utilizing the PCA device (i.e., method for recording constant infusion).
6. Return syringe cartridge to pharmacy with Proof of Use Sheet.

SINGLE-DOSE SPINAL ADMINISTRATION
OF PRESERVATIVE-FREE
MORPHINE SULFATE

I. General statement of purpose

    This policy and procedure provides standards of care for the management of the patient who has been given a single dose of epidural or intrathecal morphine sulfate (preservative-free) for postoperative pain relief.

II. Definition

    Epidural/intrathecal analgesia is used to provide postoperative pain control for selected patients. Proper use of a single dose of epidurally/intrathecally administered preservative-free morphine sulfate allows for early ambulation and provides excellent analgesia of approximately 12–18 hr in duration.

III. Guidelines

    A. This policy and procedure shall apply only to adult patients:
        1. Postoperatively
        2. Who have been given a single dose of epidural or intrathecal morphine sulfate

    B. Only the anesthesiologist may administer single doses of epidural or intrathecal morphine sulfate (preservative-free).

    C. SYSTEMIC CONTROLLED SUBSTANCES OR SEDATIVES MAY NOT BE GIVEN FOR 24 HR FOLLOWING PRESERVATIVE-FREE MORPHINE SULFATE ADMINISTRATION WITHOUT CONSULTING THE ACUTE PAIN SERVICE PHYSICIAN

    D. Two ampules of naloxone hydrochloride (Narcan 0.4 mg/ml) will be available, in the event that reversal of the effects of the morphine becomes necessary.

    E. Patients who have received spinal morphine are to be closely monitored for somnolence and respiratory depression.

    F. Nonsterile disposable gloves should be worn when manipulating or removing the epidural catheter.

    G. Before providing care to a patient who has received a single bolus injection of spinal morphine, all nursing personnel must attend inservice classes provided by the Department of Anesthesiology/Nursing Education Department.

IV. Responsibilities

    A. Anesthesiologist
        1. Explains the risks, benefits and potential complications to the patient and documents this in the "History and Progress Notes."

2. Administers the morphine sulfate (preservative-free) and records the dose and time administered on the "Anesthesia" or "PAR record," and the "Pain Service Consult Note"
3. Notifies the acute pain physician that the patient has received epidural intrathecal preservative-free morphine sulfate
4. Writes prescriptions which include the following:
    a. Route, dose, and time morphine administered
    b. The availability of naloxone hydrochloride
    c. Antiemetic therapy to be administered
    d. Frequency and parameters of respiratory and sedation level assessment
    e. Head of bed elevation >30°
5. Determines the need for additional monitoring (apnea monitor/pulse oximetry) and if indicated, writes the order

B. Registered Nurse
    1. Verifies the presence of a complete written prescription on the "Doctor's Order Sheet"
    2. Maintains a patent intravenous catheter or heparin lock for a minimum of 24 hr following morphine administration
    3. Has knowledge of the following:
        a. Risks/benefits and potential complications of epidural/intrathecal administration of morphine sulfate
        b. Pharmacology of drug administered
        c. Immediate and long-term side effects of morphine sulfate and intervention(s) to be taken if they occur
    4. Has current Basic Life Support certification
    5. Knows how to contact the APS Resident physician
    6. Confirms the presence of naloxone hydrochloride in the patient's unit dose cassette
    7. Monitors patient and documents patient response
    8. Documents nursing interventions
    9. Notifies APS physician if patient exhibits any of the following:
        a. Respiratory rate of <10 breaths/min
        b. Somnolence or confusion
        c. Hypotension
        d. Pruritus
        e. Urinary retention
    10. Assures that head of bed is elevated >30°
    11. Places apnea monitor/pulse oximeter on patient if prescribed
    12. Administers prophylactic naloxone hydrochloride as prescribed

13. Consults with APS Clinical Nurse Coordinator when necessary
V. Monitoring
   A. Note and record on the "Daily Patient Care Record" the patient's respiratory rate every hour for the first 24 hr.
   B. Assesses the patient every 4 hr for the first 24 hr:
      1. Level of sedation
      2. Blood pressure
   C. Assesses the patient at least every shift for the first 24 hr for:
      1. Pruritus
      2. Urinary retention
      3. Nausea and vomiting
      4. Adequacy of pain relief

CONTINUOUS EPIDURAL INFUSIONS FOR POSTOPERATIVE ANALGESIA: POLICY I

I. General statement of purpose
   This policy and procedure provides standards of care for the management of patients receiving epidural controlled substances, through a temporary indwelling epidural catheter, either by intermittent bolus or a continuous infusion.
II. Definition
   Epidural analgesia is used to provide postoperative pain control for selected patients. Proper use of epidural analgesia via intermittent bolus or continuous infusion allows for early ambulation, improvement of pulmonary function, increased ability to cough and clear secretions, and patient comfort.
III. Guidelines
   A. SYSTEMIC CONTROLLED SUBSTANCES OR SEDATIVES SHALL NOT BE GIVEN WITHOUT NOTIFYING THE ACUTE PAIN SERVICE.
   B. Epidural analgesics are to be administered by the Acute Pain Service physician. (S)he is responsible for the administration of the intermittent boluses as needed or initiation of the continuous epidural infusion.
   C. Two ampules of naloxone hydrochloride (Narcan 0.4 mg/ml) should be available, should reversal of the side effects of the epidural opioid be necessary.
   D. Nonsterile disposable gloves shall be worn when manipulating or removing the epidural catheter.
   E. The epidural catheter is to be manipulated or removed by the APS physician.

  F.   Nursing personnel will attend inservice classes provided by the Department of Anesthesiology/Nursing Education Department before providing care to a patient receiving epidural analgesia.

IV. Responsibilities

  A.   Department of Anesthesiology

     1.   Explains and documents in "History and Progress Notes" the risks/benefits and potential complications to the patient.

     2.   Inserts the epidural catheter, secures the epidural catheter, and labels the epidural catheter.

     3.   Writes a prescription which shall include:

        a.   For intermittent bolus: medication, dose, route, and time administered

        b.   For continuous infusion: solution, concentration of medication(s), route of administration, rate of infusion, and time initiated

        c.   The availability of naloxone hydrochloride

        d.   Antiemetic to be administered if needed

        e.   Frequency and parameters of respiratory and sedation level assessment

        f.   Elevation of the head of bed

     4.   Administers the intermittent opioid bolus or initiates a continuous opioid infusion via the epidural catheter.

     5.   Performs and documents all catheter manipulations.

     6.   Determines need for pulse oximetry/apnea monitoring and instructs nursing personnel on proper use.

     7.   Assures that consulting service house officer has knowledge of epidural drug administration.

     8.   Records controlled substance administered on "Anesthesia" or "PAR Record" and/or "Pain Service Consult Note."

     9.   Removes epidural catheter upon completion of therapy.

  B.   Nursing

     1.   Verifies the presence of a completed written prescription on the "Doctor's Order Sheet."

     2.   Maintains a patent intravenous catheter or heparin lock for a minimum of 24 hr following epidural bolus injection or while a continuous epidural infusion is in progress.

     3.   Has knowledge of the following:

        a.   Risks/complications and benefits of epidural analgesics

        b.   Pharmacology of analgesic agents administered

        c.   Immediate and long-term side effects of the opioids/ local anesthetics being utilized and nursing intervention(s) to be taken should they occur

4. Has Basic Life Support certification.
5. Knows how to contact the Acute Pain Service Resident physician.
6. Confirms the presence of naloxone hydrochloride in the patient's unit dose cassette.
7. Records required information on controlled substance Proof of Use Sheet.
8. Monitors patient and documents patient's response to therapy.
9. Notifies Acute Pain Service physician if the patient exhibits any of the following:
   a. Respiratory rate of <10 breaths/min
   b. Somnolence or confusion
   c. Hypotension
   d. Pruritus
   e. Urinary retention
10. Assures head of bed elevation is as prescribed.
11. Places apnea monitor/pulse oximeter on patient if prescribed.
12. Administers naloxone hydrochloride as required and documents its administration.
13. Discards, in the presence of a witness, the remainder of the epidural infusion solution upon discontinuing the infusion or changing the solution.
14. Consults with APS Clinical Coordinator when necessary.

V. Monitoring
   A. Notes and record on the "Critical Care Record"/"Daily Patient Care Record" the patient's respiratory rate and blood pressure every hour while receiving epidural analgesia.
   B. Assesses and documents on the "Critical Care Record"/"Daily Patient Care Record" the patient's level of sedation every 2 hr × 4, then every 4 hr while receiving epidural analgesics.
   C. Assesses the patient every shift while (s)he is receiving epidural analgesias for the following:
      1. Nausea and vomiting
      2. Urinary retention
      3. Signs and symptoms of infection
      4. Leakage at the epidural catheter insertion site
      5. Pruritus
      6. Response to pain therapy
   D. Assesses patient every shift for skin breakdown, and sensory/motor deficits if local anesthetics are added to the epidural opioid solution.

DIVISION OF NURSING PROCEDURE FOR
MAINTAINING EPIDURAL CATHETERS: POLICY II
(ADAPTED FROM EMORY UNIVERSITY HOSPITAL)

Purpose: To provide continuous site-specific pain relief for the patient experiencing acute or chronic pain.

Equipment: IMED Pump, Accuset Closed System, Y-Administration set, and epidural solution with preservative-free medication(s).

Procedure	Key points/rationale
1. Establish IV access.	
2. The epidural catheter is inserted, the patient is placed on the IMED pump by the anesthesiology staff, and the initial bolus is given and the rate is set by the APS.	Micron filter may be omitted if it obstructs flow. If pump alarms "occlusion," the catheter may be kinked. Notify APS immediately.
3. Tape over any injection ports on IV tubing with adhesive tape.	*Do not give any other solutions or medications through the epidural catheter.*
4. Label IMED pump, IV tubing, and patient's chart "EPIDURAL."	Due to the risk of respiratory depression, *No* opioids or sedatives (including anti-emetics, antipruritics and sleeping pills) may be given to a patient receiving epidural opioids without the permission of an APS physician.
5. The APS physician may give a bolus dose of concentrated local anesthetic to check the position of the epidural catheter.	After this bolus the physician will check the patient for signs of intravenous injection (dizziness, tinnitus, circumoral numbness or increase in heart rate) or subarachnoid injection (widespread numbness or weakness, fall in blood pressure).
6. A subsequent bolus dose may be given by the nurse if ordered, as follows: a. Establish location and pain. b. Check vital signs.	If the patient complains of pain, the infusion rate may be inadequate and should be adjusted as ordered by the APS. This usually involves a bolus dose

c. Check for weakness or numbness (especially in the legs).

7. If a bolus is ordered:
   a. Set "volume to be infused" on the IMED pump to equal the volume ordered (e.g., 10 ml).
   b. Increase IMED rate to 299 ml/hr.
   c. Infuse ordered bolus at this rate.
   d. Reset IMED to previous rate.
   e. Reset "volume to be infused."

and/or an upward adjustment of rate.

10 ml will infuse in approximately 2 min. The nurse must remain with the patient throughout this procedure. If the patient complains of pain, stop the bolus and call APS.

8. Check blood pressure and respiratory rate at 10, 20, and 30 min after the bolus is given.

9. Check patency of epidural catheter if ordered.
   a. Aspirate 2 ml of *preservative-free* normal saline into a 3-ml syringe.
   b. Disconnect IMED tubing from epidural catheter.
   c. Cap IMED tubing with a sterile cap or sterile needle.
   d. Attach the syringe containing the preservative-free normal saline to epidural catheter connector.
   e. Aspirate catheter. If no fluid returns, continue procedure.
   f. Inject *preservative-free* saline through epidural catheter.
   g. Reconnect epidural catheter to IMED tubing.
   h. Re-start IMED.

The normal saline used to flush an epidural catheter must be *preservative free* (10 ml single dose vial). Small amounts of air (<3–4 cc) in the epidural catheter are harmless. If fluid or blood is aspirated from epidural catheter, stop the procedure and call APS. If unable to flush catheter, call APS.

Monitoring

1. Check patients receiving epidural opioids q 1 hr × 24 hr for:

Decreased level of consciousness (LOC) reported immediately to APS physician.

a. Level of consciousness.
b. Respiratory rate.
c. Blood pressure.
Vital signs thereafter, q 4 hr until 24 hr after removal of epidural catheter.

2. Check patients receiving epidural *local anesthetics only* q 4 hr for:
   a. Blood pressure (lying and sitting when ambulatory).
   b. Analgesic level.
   c. Motor strength.

   Hypotension, somnolence, respiratory depression, motor weakness, extensive sensory anesthesia should be reported immediately to the APS physician. Emergencies may be handled by the in-house anesthesia house office.

3. Check dressing q shift. *Do not change.* Loose dressing should be reinforced with tape and physician notified.

4. Check tubing every shift. Do not reconnect if tubing becomes dislodged. Cap the line and notify APS.

   Do not clamp or kink tubing.

5. Check for urinary retention q 4 hr.

   Call APS for inability to void.

6. Check LOC q 4 hr

   Call APS immediately if patient is excessively sleepy.

7. Change IMED tubing q 48 hr.

   Epidural infusions must always be delivered by a volumetric (IMED) pump.

8. Change epidural infusion bag at least q 24 hr.

9. Maintain IV access for 24 hr after removal of epidural catheter.

All members of the APS will make rounds at least q 24 hr to assess the patient and catheter function.

Call APS for: (a) pain at insertion site; and (b) fever of >101°; and (c) catheter becoming dislodged (any manipulation of the epidural catheter should be performed by the APS).

Patient teaching: (a) Inform patient he/she may not shower or take a tub bath while epidural catheter is in place. (b) Instruct patient to call for assistance when getting out of bed. (This is to protect the catheter and dressing from becoming dislodged.) (c) Instruct patient to report: nausea and vomiting; itching; or numbness or weakness in legs. (d) Patients may ambulate as ordered by the surgeon.

INTERPLEURAL ANALGESIA FOR POSTOPERATIVE ANALGESIA AND CHRONIC PAIN MANAGEMENT

I. General statement of purpose

    This policy and procedure provides standards of care for the management of patients receiving interpleural analgesia through a temporary indwelling interpleural catheter, either by intermittent bolus or continuous infusion.

II. Definition

    Interpleural analgesia is used to provide postoperative and chronic pain control for selected patients. Proper use of interpleural analgesia via intermittent bolus or continuous infusion allows for early ambulation, improved pulmonary function, increased ability to cough and clear secretions, decreased control substance administration, and patient comfort.

III. Guidelines

    A. SYSTEMIC CONTROLLED SUBSTANCES OR SEDATIVES SHALL NOT BE GIVEN WITHOUT NOTIFYING THE ACUTE PAIN SERVICE.

    B. Interpleural analgesics shall be administered by the Acute Pain Service physician who is responsible for administering the intermittent bolus as needed or initiating the continuous interpleural infusion.

    C. Nonsterile disposable gloves are to be worn when manipulating or removing the epidural catheter.

    D. The interpleural catheter is to be removed or manipulated only by the Acute Pain Service physician.

    E. A chest x-ray shall be taken within 1 hr of insertion and within 24 hr of removal.

    F. Nursing personnel must attend inservice classes provided by the Department of Anesthesiology before providing care to a patient receiving interpleural analgesia.

IV. Responsibilities

    A. APS Physician, Department of Anesthesiology

        1. Explain to the patient and document in "History and Progress Notes" the potential risks/benefits and complications.

2. Insert, properly secure and label the interpleural catheter.
3. Should ensure that a chest x-ray is taken within 1 hr after insertion and within 24 hr after removal of the catheter.
4. Write orders which should include:
   a. For intermittent bolus: local anesthetic, dose, route, and time to be administered.
   b. For continuous infusion: solution, concentration of local anesthetic, route of administration, infusion rate and starting time.
   c. Antiemetic to be administered if needed
   d. Frequency and parameters of respiratory assessment
   e. Assess for signs of local anesthetic toxicity
      1. Parameters of heart rate
      2. Parameters of blood pressure
      3. Mental status changes
   f. No systemic opioids unless APS physician notified
5. Administer the intermittent local anesthetic bolus or initiate a continuous local anesthetic infusion via the catheter.
6. Perform and document all catheter manipulations.
7. Assure that the primary service house officer has knowledge of intrapleural analgesia.
8. Record local anesthetic administered on "Anesthesia" or "PAR Record" and/or "Pain Service Consult Note."
9. Remove the catheter when therapy is discontinued.

B. Nursing
   1. Verify the presence of a completed written prescription on the "Doctor's Order Sheet."
   2. Maintain a patent intravenous catheter or heplock while an interpleural catheter is in place.
   3. Has knowledge of the:
      a. Risks/complications and benefits of interpleural analgesia (including pneumothorax and local anesthetic toxicity)
      b. Pharmacology of analgesic agents administered
      c. Side effects of the local anesthetics being utilized and the appropriate nursing intervention(s) should they occur
   4. Have current Basic Life Support certification.
   5. Catheter insertion site must be inspected every shift for signs of infection or for a nonocclusive dressing.
   6. Nursing staff must ensure that patients do not shower with an interpleural catheter in place.
   7. Vital signs should be monitored every 15 min for 1 hr after reinjection, and per routine if a continuous infusion is used.

8. Know how to contact the APS physician.
9. Record required information on MAR record
10. Monitor patient and document patient's response and nursing interventions.
11. Notify APS physician if the patient exhibits any of the following:
    a. Respiratory rate of <10 breaths/min or >24 breaths/min
    b. Change in mental status
    c. Hypotension
    d. Bradycardia
    e. Shortness of breath
    f. Extreme sedation
12. Consult with the Clinical Nurse Coordinator when necessary.

Appendix 1.3: Guidelines (Working Document)

Guidelines are adapted from the Policy and Procedures. They are kept in the conference room or at the nursing station and are to be used as a reference tool. The difference between a Policy and Procedure, and Guideline is that guidelines are more indepth, providing definitions, giving examples (charting, VAS scales documentation, etc.) and a listing of drug incompatibilities. It is a reference tool for the bedside nurse to use on a day-to-day basis; the Policy and Procedure is the governing document, which is the broad institutional standard of care.

NURSING GUIDELINES: PATIENT CONTROLLED ANALGESIA

PCA allows for the intravenous administration of small amounts of opioids at frequent intervals, keeping blood levels of the opioid within an effective range. This avoids either excessive or inadequate levels of opioids in the blood and reduces periods of excessive sedation or ineffective pain control. When using the PCA device, a patient may, when (s)he feels pain, push a button on the device with the consequent delivery of "designated" amount of opioid into the bloodstream. The duration of pain relief is generally 10–30 min, but varies according to both the opioid used and the individual patient. Each time pain is experienced or worsens, the patient may initiate another dose.

  I. General statement of purpose: This document provides guidelines for nursing professionals who will be caring for patients on a PCA infusion device used for the delivery of opioids for acute (postoperative) and chronic (intractable) pain management ordered by the Acute Pain Service, Department of Anesthesiology. This form of administering pain medication
        a. gives the patient a sense of control over his/her pain and
        b. provides a more effective method of opioid administration.

 II. Definitions
    A. PCA dose (increment): the amount of medication (in milligrams) infused when the control button is pressed by the patient.
    B. Basal rate: the amount of medication infused per hour continuously by the device between patient-initiated doses. This dose will be ordered as milligram/hour.
    C. Delay time (lockout): the inactivation time interval (minutes) imposed by the computerized timing device between patient-initiated doses.
    D. Four-hour limit: the maximum amount of medication the patient can receive over a four hour period, governing the total amount of medication infused (basal and PCA doses combined).
    E. Bolus (loading dose): the amount of medication (mg) adminis-

tered either as a loading dose or as additional doses to supplement PCA therapy. This loading dose is administered by the Acute Pain Service physician, Certified Nurse Anesthetist, or Clinical Nurse Coordinator.

III. Guidelines

1. SYSTEMIC CONTROLLED SUBSTANCES OR SEDATIVES SHALL NOT BE GIVEN WITHOUT NOTIFICATION OF THE ACUTE PAIN SERVICE. PATIENTS MAY RECEIVE SLEEPING MEDICATION WHILE ON PCA (providing there is no basal infusion).

2. Patients who would not normally receive parenteral opioids, and those who are either physically or emotionally incapable of using the PCA device, are not suitable candidates for PCA therapy.

3. Naloxone (Narcan 0.4 mg/ml) should be available in the event that it becomes necessary to reverse the effects of the PCA opioid.

4. PCA therapy is administered intravenously by a PCA infusion device that is locked at all times. Two keys are kept for the infusion device, one with the controlled substance cabinet keys on the patient care unit and the other with the APS Physician.

5. A malfunctioning PCA infusion device is to be replaced.

6. Nonsterile, disposable gloves should be worn when manipulating or changing the intravenous catheter device.

7. Audited as Schedule II controlled substances, controlled substances for PCA are supplied in syringes and stored in the locked controlled substance cabinet.

8. Renewal prescriptions should be written every 24 hr by the physician on the APS. A complete prescription shall be written every 72 hr.

9. Antiemetics prescribed for the treatment of nausea/vomiting shall be administered by the nursing staff, and may include droperidol (Inapsine), metoclopramide (Reglan), and transderm scopolamine.

10. All nursing personnel, before providing care to patients on the PCA device, including changing the PCA syringe, must attend inservice classes given by the Department of Anesthesiology/Nursing Education Department.

IV. Responsibilities

A. APS Physician (Department of Anesthesiology)

1. Patient selection: Surgeons or other primary physicians may refer patients to the APS for pain management. It is the responsibility of the anesthesiologist, however, to deter-

mine which patient(s) are suitable for PCA. The name of the referring physician should be documented. Before initiation of PCA, the pump will be explained to the patient and a consult note written either in the History and Progress notes or on the Consult Form.

2. Prescription orders: Postoperative pain medication orders for patients on PCA therapy are written by the physician on the APS and should include information on the following:
    a. Controlled substance, milligrams/cc, basal rate, PCA increment, delay time (lockout time), and 4-hr maximum allowance of opioid
    b. Availability of naloxone (Narcan)
    c. Antiemetic(s) to be administered if needed
    d. Frequency of respirations
    e. Discontinuation of all other controlled substances and central nervous system depressants while the patient is on PCA
    f. Renewal orders should be written every 24 hr
3. Patients using PCA are to be assessed daily for level of pain relief, level of sedation, side effects and treatment, among other things, and appropriate documentation made in the history and progress notes or on follow-up progress note pages.
4. The APS physician must ensure the provision of round the clock coverage.

B. Pharmacy responsibilities
1. The supply and distribution of analgesics is the responsibility of the Department of Pharmacy Services.
2. The analgesic syringe will be dispensed by the pharmacy, as a Class II controlled substance, with an accompanying Controlled Substances Record.

C. Nursing responsibilities
1. Verifies the presence of a complete written prescription on the "Doctor's Order Sheet."
2. Maintains a patent intravenous catheter, according to established procedures (Epidemiology and Centers for Disease Control guidelines).
3. Be knowledgeable about the pharmacology of the opioids administered.
4. Knows how to contact the APS physician.
5. Confirms the availability of naloxone.
6. Upon completion of the inservice class: responsible for initiation of the PCA, changing of pump syringes, selecting appropriate controlled substance.

7. Records all necessary information on the controlled substance Proof of Use Sheet, when initiating or changing the PCA pump syringe or discontinuing PCA therapy.
8. Discards the controlled substance, in presence of a witness, on the Proof of Use Sheet. Witness must co-sign the form.
9. Records the amount of medication received by the patient through the PCA device on the medication administration record (MAR) should be done at the end of each 8 hour shift and the accumulated dose recorded in milligrams (see Appendix 1.7 for examples).
10. Monitors patients using PCA, and documents their response to therapy, as well as any nursing interventions required.
    a. Patient assessment should be done and routinely charted. Assessment includes, but is not limited to:
        i. Level of analgesia at rest and with movement: no pain, slight discomfort, mild discomfort, moderate discomfort, or severe pain.
        ii. Level of consciousness (LOC): alert, oriented, initiates conversation; drowsy, oriented, initiates conversation; drowsy, oriented, DOES NOT initiate conversation; very drowsy, disoriented, DOES NOT initiate conversation; or unresponsive, disoriented, DOES NOT initiate conversation. The PCA infusion should be stopped, and the APS Physician called immediately when LOC is equivalent to very drowsy or unresponsive.
        iii. Nursing personnel are to monitor and record intake and output, and should watch for urinary retention.
        iv. If the patient complains of nausea, or is vomiting, but has stable vital signs (i.e., patient is not bradycardiac and is normotensive), treatment should be ordered by the APS physician. If nausea/vomiting is excessive or has not improved with the prescribed antiemetic, the APS Physician should be called for further treatment.
        v. Respiratory rate is to be assessed—*as ordered by the anesthesiologist*—and charted on daily record sheets. IF THE RESPIRATORY RATE IS 10 BREATHS/MIN OR LESS, PCA

SHOULD BE STOPPED AND THE APS PHYSICIAN CALLED IMMEDIATELY.

vi. Patient assessment is to be documented in "History and Progress Notes." Examples: (a) 1/1/90, 10:00 am, Mrs. Smith remains comfortable on PCA therapy, alert with minimal pain. (b) 1/1/91, 6:00 pm, Mrs. Smith found snoring in bed at 2 pm, respiratory rate of 8. Able to arouse only by vigorous stimulation. PCA stopped. APS Physician notified. Seen by APS, Dr. Jones. PCA terminated for 2 hr, then resumed at a lower rate per physician order. Patient presently alert and awake with mild discomfort.

11. Nursing staff should possess knowledge of drug incompatibilities (see Appendix 1.9).
12. The APS Physician should be called for inadequate analgesia or for any questions or problems related to PCA.
13. The APS Clinical Nurse Coordinator should be called for clinical consultation as needed.

EPIDURAL ANALGESIA

Epidural analgesia is employed to provide postoperative pain control for selected patients. Use of epidural narcotics permits early ambulation, improvement of pulmonary function with increased ability to cough and clear secretions, and improved patient comfort.

I. General statement of purpose: This document provides guidelines for nursing professionals involved in the care of patients receiving epidural opioids, by either intermittent bolus or continuous infusion.

II. Guidelines

1. These guidelines shall apply only to patients who are receiving epidural opioids (preservative free morphine, fentanyl, meperidine or sufentanil) either by intermittent bolus or continuous infusion through an epidural catheter.
2. SYSTEMIC CONTROLLED SUBSTANCES OR SEDATIVES SHALL NOT BE ADMINISTERED WITHOUT NOTIFICATION OF THE APS.
3. The APS physician is responsible for the administration of epidural analgesics, initiating the continuous epidural infusion, or administering the intermittent bolus as needed.
4. Naloxone, 2 ampules (Narcan 0.4 mg/ml each), are to be available should reversal of the side effects of the epidural opioid be necessary.

5. When manipulating or removing the epidural catheter, nonsterile disposable gloves should be worn.

6. All patients receiving epidural analgesia must have a patent intravenous catheter or heparin lock in place until 24 hr after the last dose of opioid administered through the epidural catheter or until the continuous infusion is discontinued.

7. Patients receiving epidural analgesia must be monitored closely for somnolence and respiratory depression. Respiratory rate/depth should be assessed hourly for the first 24 hr postoperatively and documented. Sedation is to be assessed every 2 hr for the first 4 hr, and then every 4 hr postoperatively, and documented. Level of analgesia is to be assessed and documented every shift.

8. The anesthesiologist determines which patient(s), if any, require monitoring with an apnea monitor or pulse oximeter. The following patients are considered to be at greater risk for respiratory depression from epidural opioids:
   a. Individuals over 50 years of age
   b. Patients with moderate to severe medical diseases
   c. Patients who have received large doses of epidural opioids
   d. Patients with thoracic incisions
   e. Patients who have prolonged surgery
   f. Patients with history of COPD
   g. Patients receiving concomitant parenteral opioids

9. To prevent inadvertent epidural administration of solutions/medications intended for intravenous use, the epidural catheter will be clearly identified with a preprinted label and injection ports taped over.

10. An epidural catheter may remain in place for up to five days, provided the patient does not develop a temperature over 101°. Although epidural opioids may, by their own action, raise the patient's basal temperature by 1°F, the increase is gradual and steady rather than sudden and sharp. In temperatures above 101° benefits of therapy versus risk of infection must be weighed on a case by case basis to determine whether the catheter should be removed.

11. The catheter insertion sites of patients whose temperatures are elevated should be assessed, and culture and sensitivity taken if purulent drainage is noted. The anesthesiologist must be notified and the epidural catheter discontinued.

12. Leaking epidural catheters
    a. If an epidural catheter is leaking but not disconnected at the connector site, its connector may be changed using sterile technique

      b.   If an epidural catheter is disconnected at the connector site and contaminated, the catheter should be discontinued by the anesthesiologist

      c.   If an epidural catheter is leaking at the insertion site, the catheter should be evaluated by the anesthesiologist

13.   The epidural catheter may remain in place for patients started on Coumadin after its placement. Patients who are started on intermittent heparin therapy may continue to receive epidural analgesia. If a continuous heparin infusion is to be started, the anesthesiologist must be notified to discontinue the epidural catheter prior to the initiation of heparin therapy.

14.   Nursing personnel are required to attend inservice classes provided by the Department of Anesthesiology/Nursing Education Department before they provide care to a patient receiving epidural analgesia.

15.   The Clinical Nurse Coordinator should be called for clinical consultation as needed.

III. Responsibilities

    A.   Acute pain physician (Department of Anesthesiology)

        1.   It will be determined during the preoperative visit or initial consultative visit, whether or not a patient is a suitable candidate for epidural analgesia. Patients may be referred to the APS for pain management by surgeons and other primary physicians. However, the anesthesiologist is the individual responsible for determining which patient(s) will be suitable for epidural opioids. The anesthesiologist also assumes responsibility for the placement of the catheter and the management of all analgesics, including systemic analgesics.

        2.   All potential risks and complications of epidural analgesia will be discussed with the patient by the anesthesiologist and will be documented in the History and Progress notes or on the Consult Form.

        3.   The anesthesiologist is responsible for inserting, properly securing and labeling the epidural catheter.

        4.   To facilitate postoperative follow up, the catheter should be covered at the insertion site using a transparent dressing (e.g., TEGADERM), and should be securely taped to the back and properly labeled. A cap should be placed at the catheter's injection port when intermittent boluses are to be administered to ensure sterility. If a patient is on a continuous epidural infusion, all injection ports must be covered to avoid inadvertent administration of solutions/medications into the epidural catheter. Catheter is labeled

"EPIDURAL." NO MEDICATION OTHER THAN THE OPIOID AND/OR OPIOID/LOCAL MIXTURE IS TO BE ADMINISTERED THROUGH THE EPIDURAL CATHETER.

5. Postoperative orders are to be written by the anesthesiologist and should include the following:
   a. No systemic opioids to be given
   b. For intermittent bolus doses: drug, dose and time administered
   c. For infusion: drug(s) and rate of infusion if patient is receiving a continuous epidural opioid infusion
   d. Frequency of assessment of respiratory rate and level of sedation
   e. Level of analgesia assessed and documented every shift
   f. Head of bed >30°
   g. Parameters for O_2 saturation if pulse oximetry is used
   h. Parameters for respiratory rate and treatment of respiratory depression
   i. Nausea/vomiting, if indicated
   j. Treatment for pruritus (itching)
   k. Treatment for urinary retention
   l. Naloxone, 2 ampules (Narcan 0.4 mg/ml), should be at bedside

6. The anesthesiologist administers the drug(s) to patients receiving intermittent boluses of epidural opioids. The response is closely monitored by the nursing staff. The anesthesiologist remains with the patient until a satisfactory response is achieved.

7. For patients on a continuous infusion (either opioid or opioid/local anesthetic), the anesthesiologist (in addition to the nursing staff), is responsible for assessing the patient's response to the therapy: i.e., level of analgesia and level of sedation, and when necessary, should make appropriate changes in therapy.

8. When preparing the medication for intermittent bolus/continuous epidural infusion, the amount of controlled substance remaining must be discarded in the presence of a witness (Registered Nurse).

9. The Anesthesiologist is responsible for determining which patients will require apnea monitoring or pulse oximetry.

10. All catheter manipulations (i.e., intermittent doses, removal), will be performed by the anesthesiologist and documented in the patient's record.

11. Responsible for ordering naloxone as needed, its administration and documentation.

12. Patients receiving epidural opioids are to be assessed daily by the anesthesiologist, and the following noted in the history and progress notes, or follow-up progress notes: level of pain relief, level of sedation, appearance of catheter insertion site, side effects and treatments.

13. Provision should be made for round the clock coverage.

B. Nursing personnel

1. Verify the presence of a completed written prescription on the "Doctor's Order Sheet."

2. Maintain a patent intravenous or heparin lock until 24 hours after administration of the last intermittent dose of epidural opioid or while the patient is receiving a continous opioid infusion.

3. Has knowledge of the pharmacology of analgesic agents employed, the immediate and long-term side effects of the controlled substances/local anesthetics, and appropriate nursing intervention(s) should they occur.

4. Confirm the availability of naloxone (Narcan 0.4 mg/ml) in the patient's unit dose cassette.

5. Know how to contact the APS Resident physician.

6. Record necessary information on controlled substance Proof of Use Sheet.

7. Discard, in the presence of a witness, the remaining epidural infusion solution, when discontinuing an infusion or changing the solution container. Both individuals must sign the "Proof of Use" record.

8. Monitor rate and depth of the patient's respirations every hour for the first 24 hr.

9. Monitors patient's level of sedation every 2 hr for the first 4 hr; then every 4 hr. Level of sedation: Alert, oriented, initiates conversation; drowsy, oriented, initiates conversation; drowsy, oriented, *does not* initiate conversation; very drowsy, disoriented, *does not* initiate conversation; stupor, disoriented, *does not* initiate conversation.

10. Assess and document patient's level of analgesia every shift. Level of analgesia at rest and with movement: no pain; slight discomfort; mild discomfort; moderate discomfort; and severe pain.

11. Monitor intake and output for 24 hr. APS should be notified for urinary retention.

12. Treat pruritus as ordered. Pruritus is a common side effect of epidural opioids, usually occurring on the face, head,

and neck. Skin conditions such as rash, urticaria, and wheals are not normal side effects of epidural opioids.

13. Nausea and vomiting occurs in about 50% of the patients receiving epidural opioids. Treatment is to be determined by the APS Physician and may include droperidol, metoclopramide, and transdermal Scopolamine.

14. The following steps should be taken if respiratory depression should occur:
    a. Assess patient's level of sedation. Patient may be stimulated to take a breath.
    b. Treat respiratory depression with naloxone (Narcan), as ordered by the anesthesiologist and/or APS physician.
    c. Notify APS physician immediately.
    d. If apnea occurs, support respiration by using ambu bag and mask ventilation until the patient can be assessed by the APS physician.

15. Reinforce tape as needed to maintain the catheter. If catheter is inadvertently dislodged, a dry sterile dressing should be placed at the catheter insertion site, the catheter saved, and the APS physician notified.

16. Check catheter insertion site for redness, swelling, purulent drainage. Notify the APS physician if there is any sign of infection.

17. Monitor epidural catheters for leakage:
    a. If leaking at connector site but not disconnected, may change connector using sterile technique.
    b. If an epidural catheter becomes disconnected from connector and contaminated, the catheter should be discontinued.
    c. If an epidural catheter is leaking at the insertion site, the catheter should be evaluated by the Anesthesiologist.

18. Monitor patient for postural hypotension (i.e., when the head of the bed is elevated, when the patient dangles at the side of the bed, or when the patient ambulates for the first time). Systemic vascular resistance may be lowered by the opioid, particularly in the presence of intravascular fluid depletion.

19. Place patient on apnea monitor or pulse oximeter if ordered. The APS Physician is to be notified if O_2 saturation is <90%.

20. For patients who have had a local anesthetic combined with the opioid, the nurse should monitor patient for:

      a.   Hypotension (due to venous pooling and peripheral vascular resistance)

      b.   Bradycardia (due to blockade of the cardiac accelerator nerves).

      c.   Decreased cutaneous sensation (may increase the risk of skin breakdown).

      d.   Extensive motor block (could result in respiratory insufficiency and may be secondary to migration of the catheter into the subarachnoid space).

21.   If the patient reports or exhibits behavioral signs of continued pain, the APS physician should be notified.

22.   Consult with APS Clinical Nurse Coordinator, as indicated.

DIFFERENTIATING EPIDURAL ANESTHESIA FROM ANALGESIA

Type	Characteristics
Anesthesia	Blocks conduction in both sensory and motor nerves producing loss of both sensory and motor function. Drugs that may be used: 2% lidocaine; 0.5% bupivacaine.
Analgesia	Motor and sensory function preserved; selective blockade of nociceptive action potential; alterations of pain transmission at the dorsal horn. Drugs used: opioids; dilute local anesthetic solutions

Surgical anesthesia is provided by the injection of local anesthetics into the epidural space, in relatively high concentrations and large volumes. The same effect may be achieved by the injection of considerably smaller doses injected into the subarachnoid space. Both block nerve conduction in sensory, motor and sympathetic nerves, resulting in lack of sensation, paralysis, vasodilatation. Lower concentrations and smaller volumes of epidural local anesthetics provide pain relief and sympathetic blockade without significant motor nerve blockade. Very dilute local anesthetic solutions provide selective pain relief (via c-fiber blockade) without other affects.

The provision of pain relief is the primary goal of epidural local anesthetic use outside the operating room.

Dilute solutions of local anesthetics are used for analgesia to block sensory fibers (specifically pain fibers), yet spare motor fibers. When added to epidural opioid infusions, the local anesthetic enhances the effect of the opioid. Thus, decreasing the total opioid dose requirement and reducing untoward side effects.

PHYSIOLOGY OF PAIN

1. Pain fibers enter the dorsal horn of the spinal cord and synapse with second order neurons in the area known as the substantia gelatinosa. The ascending fibers carry the "pain" message to the thalamus and cerebral cortex where it is interpreted as such.
2. The neuropeptides including substance P, are believed to mediate nociceptive transmission.
3. Opiate receptors are also located in the dorsal horn of the spinal cord. When opiates bind with receptors, the release of substance P is blocked, thus altering the transmission and subsequent perception of pain.

OPIOIDS COMMONLY USED FOR EPIDURAL ANALGESIA

Although preparations of morphine and hydromorphone are FDA approved for epidural use, preservative-free solutions of fentanyl, sufentanil, meperidine, and methadone have also been successfully employed. Epidurally administered opioids may be combined with dilute solutions of local anesthetics, usually 0.1% bupivacaine.

DISTRIBUTION OF EPIDURAL OPIOIDS

Location	Characteristics
Vascular uptake	Plasma concentrations resemble those following an intramuscular dose
CSF	CSF concentrations rise slowly but may remain elevated for up to 20 hr with hydrophilic opioids such as morphine
Spinal cord	Opioids bind and activate opioid receptors in the substantia gelatinosa
Extradural fat	Large surface area for uptake of drugs, especially those which are highly lipophilic

INTERPLEURAL ANALGESIA

Interpleural analgesia is a recently developed technique of pain relief, suitable for both acute postoperative pain, as well as chronic pain management. The technique involves the percutaneous placement of a flexible catheter via a thin walled Tuohy needle into the interpleural space. The catheter may be placed in the operating room at the end of surgery, in the PACU, in the ICU or in the patient's room.

Interpleural analgesia is particularly, but not exclusively, indicated for patients who would be at more than the usual risk for postoperative respiratory insufficiency. This being either due to ventilatory insufficiency secondary to postoperative pain, opioid-induced ventilatory depression, or particular patient characteristics that would make one more likely to incur postoperative respiratory insufficiency (e.g., CHF, COPD, morbid obesity).

I. General statement of purpose: This document provides guidelines for nursing professionals who will be caring for patients receiving interpleural analgesia, either by intermittent bolus or a continuous infusion. Indications for interpleural analgesia: (a) cholecystectomy, (b) unilateral breast surgery, (c) renal surgery, (d) other subcostal incisions, (e) thoracotomies, and (f) multiple rib fractures and/or flail chest.

II. Guidelines

1. This document shall apply only to patients who are receiving interpleural analgesia using local anesthetics, either in intermittent bolus or continuous infusions via an interpleural catheter.

2. SYSTEMIC CONTROLLED SUBSTANCES OR SEDATIVES SHALL NOT BE GIVEN WITHOUT NOTIFYING THE APS.

3. Interpleural analgesia shall be administered by the APS physician who shall be responsible for the administration of the intermittent bolus as needed or initiation and maintenance of a continuous interpleural infusion.

4. Nonsterile disposable gloves shall be worn when manipulating or removing the catheter.

5. All patients receiving interpleural analgesia must have a patent intravenous catheter or heparin lock in place until the interpleural catheter is removed.

6. Patients receiving interpleural analgesia must be monitored closely for somnolence, local anesthetic toxicity, and respiratory complications.

   a. Breath sounds shall be evaluated at least every shift.

   b. Level of consciousness shall be evaluated every four hours.

   c. Level of analgesia will be assessed and charted every shift.

7. The interpleural catheter must be clearly identified, using a pre-

printed label to prevent inadvertent administration of solutions/ medications into the interpleural space.

8. The interpleural catheter may remain in place up to five days, providing that there is no elevation in temperature above 101.5°.

9. If patient has an elevated temperature, assess the insertion site. If purulent drainage is noted, culture and sensitivity should be taken. The anesthesiologist must be notified and the interpleural catheter should be discontinued.

10. Leaking interpleural catheters.
     a. Interpleural catheters leaking at the connector site, but not disconnected, may have connector changing using sterile technique
     b. Interpleural catheters disconnected from the connector and contaminated will be discontinued
     c. Interpleural catheters leaking at the insertion site should be evaluated by the anesthesiologist

11. Nursing personnel should attend inservice classes provided by the Department of Anesthesiology/Nursing Education Department before providing care to a patient receiving interpleural analgesia.

12. For clinical consultation, call the Clinical Nurse Coordinator as needed.

III. Responsibilities
   A. Acute Pain Physician (Department of Anesthesiology)
       1. At the time of the preoperative or initial consultative visit, it will be determined if the patient is a candidate for interpleural analgesia. Surgeons or other primary physicians may refer patients to the Acute Pain Service for pain management. However, it will be the responsibility of the anesthesiologist to determine which patient(s) will be suitable for interpleural analgesia. The anesthesiologist assumes responsiblity for placement of the catheter and management of all analgesics for the patient, including systemic analgesics. Contraindications: (a) PEEP; (b) pleural fibrosis, pleural adhesions, pleuritis; (c) pleural effusion; (d) infection at proposed site of insertions; (e) allergy to the intended local anesthetic; (f) bullous emphysema; (g) bleeding diatheses; and (h) recent pulmonary infection.
       3. The anesthesiologist should discuss with the patient all potential risks and complications from the interpleural catheter placement and will document in the History and Progress notes or on the Consult Form. Complications: (a) pneumothorax; (b) tension pneumothorax; (c) laceration of

intercostal vessels; (d) allergic reaction to local anesthetics; (e) local anesthetic toxicity; (f) infection; and (g) broncho-pleural fistula.

4. The anesthesiologist should insert, secure, and label the catheter clearly as "Intrapleural Catheter."

5. A transparent dressing, e.g., TEGADERM, will be used to cover the catheter at the insertion site to facilitate follow-up. The catheter will be taped securely to the patient's skin and labelled properly. The interpleural catheter will have a cap at the injection port to ensure sterility if intermittent boluses are to be given. If a patient is on a continuous infusion, the anesthesiologist must insure that all injection ports are properly covered so that inadvertent accidental administration of solutions/medications will not be injected into the interpleural catheter. NO MEDICATION IS EVER TO BE ADMINISTERED THROUGH THE INJECTION PORT OTHER THAN THE LOCAL ANESTHETIC MIXTURE.

6. Anesthesiologist will write postoperative orders. These orders should include, but are not limited to,
    a. Parameters for respiratory rate
    b. Parameters for blood pressure
    c. Parameters of heart rate
    d. Systemic opioids that may be administered for break-through pain, if necessary
    e. For intermittent bolus: local anesthetic, dose (concentration and volume) and time given
    f. For continuous infusions: drug, concentration, and rate of infusion
    g. Chest X-ray within 1 hr of catheter insertion and within 24 hr of interpleural catheter removal

7. If the patient is receiving intermittent boluses of local anesthetic, the anesthesiologist will administer the drug. The patient's response is to be closely monitored by the nursing staff. The anesthesiologist will stay with the patient until a satisfactory response is achieved.

8. If the patient is on a continuous infusion, the anesthesiologist (in addition to the nursing staff) will be responsible for assessment of the patient's response to the therapy: i.e., level of analgesia and level of sedation. The anesthesiologist shall make appropriate changes in therapy as needed.

9. All catheter manipulations (intermittent boluses, catheter removal) must be performed and documented in the patient's hospital record by the anesthesiologist.

10. There is to be a daily assessment of the patient which is

documented in the history and progress notes or on follow-up progress notes. Assessment should include: level of pain relief, level of sedation, appearance of catheter insertion site, side effects and treatments.

11. Provide round the clock coverage.

B. Nursing personnel

1. Verify the presence of a completed written prescription on the "Doctor's Order Sheet"

2. Maintain a patent intravenous or heparin lock while the interpleural catheter is in place.

3. Has knowledge of pharmacology of local anesthetic agents administered and immediate and long-term side effects of the drugs being utilized and nursing intervention(s) to be taken if side effects occur.

4. Know how to contact the APS physician.

5. Monitor and record breath sounds, and rate and depth of respirations. Shortness of breath, increased respiratory rate, decreased or unilateral breath sounds may be indicative of a pneumothorax. Respiratory rates should be done, and lung oscillation should be performed at least once per shift.

6. Assess and document the patient's sedation level. Level of sedation: alert, oriented, initiates conversation; drowsy, oriented, initiates conversation; drowsy, oriented, *does not* initiate conversation; very drowsy, disoriented, *does not* initiate conversation; stupor, disoriented, *does not* initiate conversation.

7. Assess and document patient's level of analgesia every shift. Level of analgesia: no pain; slight discomfort; mild discomfort; moderate discomfort; severe pain.

8. Monitor for systemic toxicity: vital signs and mental status should be documented every four hours while the interpleural catheter is in place.

9. Monitor for breakthrough pain. If the patient is receiving intermittent bolus administration of a local anesthetic, the duration of analgesia should be approximately 8 hr (if bupivacaine is utilized). It is imperative that the patient be positioned correctly after the injection to obtain the desired effect of the block. The patient should be supine or with the "affected side down" for 20–30 min after injection (see Chapter 10).

     If the patient is receiving a continuous infusion, constant analgesia is the desired result. It is possible that "breakthrough" pain may occur. If this happens, positioning the patient on his/her side may allow the local anesthetic to bathe the affected area, thus reducing or eliminating the pain. The patient may require a supplemental bolus of IV/IM medication if repositioning is not effective. Patients who have a history of substance abuse, may have difficulty obtaining adequate pain relief with interpleural analgesia alone. Supplementation with parenteral opioids for these patients may be necessary.

10. Reinforce tape as needed to maintain catheter. If the catheter is inadvertently dislodged, place an occlusive dressing at the insertion site, save the catheter, and call the APS physician.

11. Check catheter's insertion site for redness, swelling, purulent drainage. Notify APS physician if any sign of infection is present.

12. Monitor catheters for leakage. Notify the APS physician if leakage is noticed.

13. Monitor patient for postural hypotension.

14. Consult with the Clinical Nurse Coordinator, as necessary.

Appendix 1.4: Credentialling

**EMORY UNIVERSITY HOSPITAL,
DIVISION OF NURSING—PROCESS OF CERTIFICATION
FOR ADVANCED NURSING SKILL:
MAINTAINING EPIDURAL CATHETERS**

Nursing units where skill is performed	Written materials available	Mediated programs
All units	"Maintaining Epidural Catheters" in Division of Nursing Procedure Manual Mini-standards on reverse side of certification slip[a] Resource person: Barbara Reed, RN, CNS, Pain Management	"New Trends in Epidural and Intrathecal Analgesia and Pain Management" 1 hr. (W0200.N4)

[a]Forms available in Nursing Quality Assurance.

Process of certification: (a) view "New Trends in Epidural and Intrathecal Analgesia and Pain Management" (W0200.N4); (b) read "Epidural Infusion of Narcotics Guidelines" and "Procedure for Maintaining Epidural Catheters"; (c) test score of 80% or higher; and (d) review documentation form for Controlled Substances.

This was approved by Directors' Conference, Division of Nursing, July 12, 1988.

**MINI-STANDARD FOR MAINTAINING
EPIDURAL CATHETERS**

RN demonstrates competency by:

1. Reviewing written and mediated materials listed in Process of Certification.

2. Achieving 80% or higher on test.
3. Demonstrating ability to use the appropriate infusion pump.
4. Verbally identifying epidural anatomy and correct catheter placement.
5. Describing analgesic action of epidural local anesthetics.
6. Describing analgesic action of epidural narcotics.
7. Discussing five most common side effects of epidural local anesthetics and narcotics.
8. Stating concentrations of three most common medications infused into an epidural catheter.
9. Stating concentrations of three most common medications infused into an epidural catheter.
10. Performing steps in catheter flushing procedure and listing actions to take if any contraindications to flushing occur.
11. Discussing patient teaching to be done for each patient with an epidural catheter in place.
12. Listing three possible complications of epidural analgesia and nursing actions to be taken.

This was approved by Directors' Conference, Division of Nursing, July 12, 1988.

EMORY UNIVERSITY HOSPITAL, DIVISION OF NURSING—CERTIFICATION FOR TECHNICAL NURSING SKILL (AS DEFINED IN CERTIFICATION POLICY)

This is the form used to certify skill:

Name _____   Procedure: *Maintaining Epidural Catheters*

Social Security Number:_____ ____ _____   Department/Unit:_____

The above nurse has received direct instruction in the technique and related policies for this procedure at Emory University Hospital. The nurse has demonstrated under my supervision adequate skill and understanding of the related policies in reference to the skill being certified.

SIGNATURE OF PERSON CERTIFYING:_____

TITLE: _____

DATE: _____

5/87

Appendix 1.5: Physician Education

YNHH/YALE UNIVERSITY SCHOOL OF MEDICINE
RESIDENT EDUCATION PROCESS
DIDACTIC SCHEDULE

Goals and Objectives of the APS Rotation

1. In an academic setting, specific training in pain management should be emphasized. Residents should be able to:
   a. Distinguish pain from anxiety
   b. Determine degree of pain and evaluate effectiveness of therapy
   c. Understand the physiologic and pharmacologic basis of PCA and spinal opioid therapy
   d. Be familiar with side effects and appropriate treatments
   e. Learn appropriate responses to each pain management therapy
   f. Be familiar with pain management therapy for pediatric patients
   g. To understand pharmacologic and physiologic basis for nonopioid analgesic therapy and its application
   h. Understand guidelines set forth for pain management, i.e., available drugs, usual dosages, use of continuous (basal) infusion, etc.
2. Residents should arrive appropriately dressed for rounds (neat street clothes and clean white lab coat). Prior to beginning work rounds, a 30–45 min didactic session is presented by the attending or fellow.
3. Didactic sessions include:
   a. Basic sciences—pharmacokinetics/pharmacodynamics of opioid and non-opioid analgesics; anatomy and physiology of pain, research
   b. Pain assessment
   c. PCA—concept/management/medications
   d. Spinal analgesia—concept/management/medications and side effects/treatment
   e. Case discussions
   f. Interpleural analgesia
   g. NSAIDs
   h. Pediatric pain management
   i. Chronic pain management (use of neurolytics, progression of analgesics in chronic pain management)
4. Following the didactic session: Off-going resident sign out to the on-coming resident, attending and nurse. Sign out rounds will cover the current patient census, and problems which occurred overnight and referrals of patients to be added to the Service.
5. Rounds: Patients are evaluated individually with regard to the efficacy of therapy, side effects and management, and changes in therapy. A progress note is written, signed by the attending, and continuation/

discontinuation orders are written. The resident carries the Log Book in which (s)he records the current census and notes any changes in therapy.

6. After rounds, the attending, nurses and resident will go over the census and discuss the management of patients newly added or about to be added to the APS. Review the operating room schedule.

7. The attending will make afternoon rounds with the resident and nurse. New patients, those from ICU and those who have had therapy changes will be seen in the afternoon.

8. The anesthesiology resident will make decisions regarding patient management considered appropriate to his/her level of knowledge and training.

9. The on-call resident should always have access to the attending's phone number and beeper.

Event Protocol

1. Bloods to be drawn by resident, timed and dated:
   a. Chemistry (10 cc of blood in a red top tube)
   b. CBC (2 cc of blood in a purple top tube)
   c. Opioid level (5 cc of blood in a red top tube)
   d. Blood toxicology screening (5 cc of blood in a red top tube)
   e. Urine toxicology screening (50 ml of urine)

   THESE SAMPLES ARE TO BE *LABELLED* (WITH PATIENT'S NAME AND UNIT NUMBER) AND HAND CARRIED TO THE MEDICINE LABORATORY. THE OPIOID LEVELS AND TOXICOLOGY SCREENING SHOULD BE PLACED ON ICE (0° OR LESS) IF THE EVENT OCCURS ON AN OFF SHIFT OR ON THE WEEKEND. Please also note the name of the technician who received the samples from you.

2. Print out of the data from the PCA pump. Date, time, pump number, patient name, and unit number should be on the printout.

3. Set pump aside with a malfunction sign, so that it does not get reused until it is checked out by engineering.

4. Drug and tubing should be placed in a plastic bag and locked in the narcotic box on the patient care unit. Please notify the CNC so that the drug may be transported to pharmacy during working hours to be analyzed.

5. Please immediately notify the attending covering the service.

6. A short note which is dated and timed should be placed in the chart stating what was done—DO NOT HYPOTHESIZE ABOUT THE CAUSE OF THE EVENT.

Appendix 1.6: Patient Education

PATIENT CONTROLLED ANALGESIA THERAPY[1]

What is PCA?

PCA is a technique that enables you, the patient to give yourself pain medication, using a computerized PCA device. PCA allows you to determine when to give yourself pain medication. When you begin to feel an increase in pain, simply press the button and you will receive a small dose of pain medication through your intravenous catheter.

About the Pump

Contained in the pump is the pain medication prescribed by the Acute Pain Service. It connects directly into your intravenous (IV), and consequently, a push of the button will send a preset dose of medication into your bloodstream. Thus, you have control over when and how often you receive pain medication.

How Often Should I Press the Button?

Whenever you have an unacceptable degree of pain, or your pain medication does not seem effective, even after pushing the button, call your nurse to check the IV and the PCA pump.

Can I Give Myself Too Much Pain Medication?

No. The PCA pump is designed to give only the amount of medication prescribed at a minimum dosage interval. The pump is set by the doctor or nurse for the amount of medication to be administered each time the button is pushed within a certain time period. The amount of time between doses allows the first dose to take effect before another may be administered. It is therefore not possible to give yourself an overdose. In addition, the total amount of medication you give yourself is being recorded by the PCA device, and cannot exceed the total amount ordered by your doctor. If any problem should arise with the device, an alarm will sound on the pump thereby alerting the nurse.

---

[1]This was modified from Abbott and Bard patient education pamplets.

How Soon Will I Feel Pain Relief After I Press the Button?

Some degree of pain relief should be felt approximately 5 to 6 minutes after administration of a dose.

Are There Any Side Effects?

There are side effects, but no more than with traditional pain therapy. You may, with either method of pain therapy, feel nauseated or drowsy.

What If I Become Uncomfortable?

If your pain medication seems to have stopped working, even after pushing the button, call the nurse to check your IV and the PCA pump.

Will I Be Totally Pain Free?

No, you will not be totally pain free. Whether you receive traditional therapy (shots) or use PCA, you will feel some pain. PCA will make the pain tolerable and provide you with control in deciding when to have pain medication. While you are receiving pain medication intravenously by PCA, you will be seen frequently by the doctor (usually a resident), the APS nurse, and your staff nurse. Please ask them any questions or share any concerns you might have with them.

PAIN RELIEF BY EPIDURAL ANALGESIA

A. Epidural analgesia: The word "epidural" or "peridural" (the terms are equivalent) refers to the space that is just outside the space containing spinal fluid. Pain medications are injected into this space to provide pain relief after your surgery.
1. Is the insertion of the needle painful? The anesthesiologist will numb your skin with local anesthetic, which will sting momentarily, prior to inserting the needle. After numbing the skin, most patients feel only firm pressure. A thin plastic tube is then carefully inserted and the needle is withdrawn. Often, but not always, when the plastic tube is inserted you may feel a twinge in one or both legs, something like "hitting your funny bone." This lasts only a moment, and is a suggestion that the tube is in the right space. The tube itself is very soft and cannot be felt, even when you are lying on your back.
2. How long does the epidural catheter stay in place? The catheter

may come out directly after surgery or may stay in place five to seven days, providing that there is no postoperative infection, you are not put on medication to "thin your blood," or there is no other reason to remove the catheter.

3. How long does the medication last? The pain medication can be given two ways:
   a. Intermittently, approximately every 12 hr or sooner if you experience pain; thus pain relief lasts approximately 12 hr with each dose.
   b. Continuous infusion, which delivers a small amount of medication all the time and usually maintains a constant level of pain relief.
4. Are there any risks?
   a. The needle or the plastic tube can go into one of the blood vessels in the epidural space. If this does occur, the anesthesiologist will take out the needle or the plastic tube and insert it again.
   b. The needle can enter the spinal space where the spinal fluid circulates. This happens in 1–2% of cases, and you may have a headache for a few days afterward.
   c. Occasionally, a sensation of numbness or tingling may last for a few days or weeks afterward. Sensation usually will return to normal with no treatment other than heat and rest.
   d. There is an extremely small chance that an infection could develop. If a patient develops a fever which is related to an infection, he/she will not be offered epidural analgesia and the catheter will be removed if it is in place.
   e. If the patient has a bleeding tendency, the needle or the plastic tube could cause some bleeding in the epidural space. It is so important for the patient to tell the doctors if anyone in his/her family is known to have a bleeding problem as this may result in a severe problem if bleeding occurs in this situation.

B. Intrathecal analgesia: Your anesthesiologist may choose spinal anesthesia for your surgery and, if so, pain medication can be given at this time. With spinal anesthesia a small dose of medication is injected into the intrathecal space (the space containing the cerebrospinal fluid). The pain medication should last approximately 12–18 hr. In some cases a catheter is placed in the intrathecal space to allow further doses of pain medication to be given.
   1. How is intrathecal analgesia given? The anesthesiologist numbs the skin and inserts a very fine needle between two of the lower backbones. The needle enters the fluid-filled space which is a little deeper than the epidural space. A small amount of medica-

tion is injected and the needle is removed. You will notice almost at once that your legs and hips are becoming numb. You will not be able to move your legs. The numbness will last 1–2 hours after the surgery is completed. When the numbness wears off, because pain medication was given with the anesthetic medication, little or no pain is felt for approximately 12 hr.

2. Is there any risk?

     a. Up to 1–3% of patients may experience a headache, which will last a few days. The anesthesiologist will use the smallest possible needle which reduces the chance of headache. Drinking plenty of fluids and taking aspirin or acetaminophen can help relieve a mild headache. Other treatment is available if the headache does not respond to this treatment.

     b. Rarely, spinal anesthesia will reach a very high level, very quickly, which may make the patient feel uncomfortable. If this happens, the anesthesiologist may feel that it is best to administer general anesthesia. This would not affect the progress of a surgery or jeopardize your care.

     c. The risk of lower blood pressure, infection or bleeding are much the same as for epidural.

Appendix 1.7A: Drug Administration Record/Flowsheet

PATIENT NAME:	UNIT NUMBER	FLOOR/ROOM	PRIMARY PHYSICIAN NAME:

DRUG	STRENGTH	TYPE: PCA ___ EPIDURAL ___ INTERPLEURAL ___ OTHER(write in) ___

DATE	TIME _____ AM _____ PM	CONTROLLED SUBSTANCE SHEET	AMOUNT HUNG	NURSE SIGNATURE:

DATE	TIME _____ AM _____ PM	AMOUNT DISCARDED	NURSES SIGNATURE 1)_____ 2)_____	AMOUNT USED

Appendix 1.7B: Drug Administration Record/Flowsheet

MEDICATION Dose, dose form, route of admin., frequency	D/C Date		DATE TIME & INITIAL	DATE TIME & INITIAL	DATE TIME & INITIAL	DATE TIME & INITIAL	DATE TIME & INITIAL
		AM					
		PM					
		AM					
		PM					

Appendix 1.7C: IV Solution And PCA Pump Controlled Drug Administration Record/Flowsheet

Drug		Strength		Quantity in ml		FORM ☐ IV Solution	☐ PCA Syringe PCA Cartridge
Issued By		Received By			Nursing Unit		
Date Issued		Date Received					

PATIENT NAME	ROOM NO.	MEDICAL RECORD NO	PHYSICIAN'S NAME

DATE   TIME   AM/PM

Total volume placed into machine or hung _____ ml

Total to prime IV tubing (minus) _____ ml

Total Loading Dose Administered (if applicable) (minus) _____ ml

Anesthesiologist/RN signature _____ = _____

Total Remaining ml in syringe

Time	Dose Per Injection or cc/hr	Number of Injections	Continuous Basal Rate	Pain (0-10)	LOC (1-5)	Resp. Rate	Pupil Size (2-10MM)	RN Signature	RN Signature (2 RN signatures are required at each shift count & on transfer.)
AM/PM									
AM/PM									
AM/PM									
AM/PM TOTAL DOSE GIVEN PER SHIFT ML LEFT TO COUNT ML									
AM/PM									
AM/PM									
AM/PM TOTAL DOSE GIVEN PER SHIFT ML LEFT TO COUNT ML									
AM/PM									
AM/PM									
AM/PM TOTAL DOSE GIVEN PER SHIFT ML LEFT TO COUNT ML									
AM/PM									
AM/PM									
AM/PM TOTAL DOSE GIVEN PER SHIFT ML LEFT TO COUNT ML									
AM/PM									
AM/PM									
AM/PM TOTAL DOSE GIVEN PER SHIFT ML LEFT TO COUNT ML									
AM/PM									
AM/PM									
AM/PM TOTAL DOSE GIVEN PER SHIFT ML LEFT TO COUNT ML									

Date _____ Time _____ AM/PM TOTAL DOSE RECEIVED BY PATIENT _____ ml _____ RN Signature

Date _____ Time _____ AM/PM Amount returned to Pharmacy _____ ml _____ RN _____ RN RPh
(All wastes must be returned to pharmacy)   (2 signatures required)

Date _____ Time _____ AM/PM Amount Actually Destroyed _____ ml by _____ RPh

Destruction Witnessed by _____ RPh _____ RPh
(3 signatures required)

Appendix 1.7D: Acute Pain Service
Department of Anesthesiology
PCA Drug Administration Record/Flowsheet

Analgesic: Morphine sulfate
              1 mg/ 1 ml

PCA dose:

Delay Time:

Basal Dose:

DATE & TIME						
NEW BASAL DOSE						
NEW PCA DOSE						

Indicate change in PCA/Basal dose with next to date and time below.

DATE											
TIME											
mgs DELIVERED SINCE LAST CHECK											
RESPIRATORY RATE											
SEDATION RATING (1-5)											
ANALGESIC RATING (1-5)											

SEDATION RATING

1 = Wide awake
2 = Drowsy
3 = Dozing intermittently
4 = Awakens only when aroused
5 = Asleep at the time of charting

ANALGESIC RATING

Ask this question verbatim:
"Which of the following describes how you have felt since you were last asked?"

1 = Comfortable
2 = In mild discomfort
3 = In pain
4 = In bad pain
5 = In very bad pain
as = Asleep at time of charting

Appendix 1.7E: Acute Pain Service
Department of Anesthesiology
Epidural Solution and PCA Drug
Administration Record/Flowsheet

PCA Loading Dose								
Dose								
Lockout								
4 hr. limit								
Basal								
Total mg								
Shifts: 11-7								
7-3								
3-11								
Nausea Rx.								
REGIONAL ANALGESIA								
M.D.								

Appendix 1.7F: PCA Drug Administration Record/Flowsheet

Drug/Concentration	Time New Cartridge Inserted	Dose (Mg)	Lockout Intervals (Mins)	Basal Infusion	4-Hour Limit	Nurses Signature	Total Doses Delivered

Time			
Respiratory Rates			
Sedation Rating*			
Analgesic Rating**			

* Sedating Rating Scale

1 = Wide awake
2 = Drowsy
3 = Dozing intermittently
4 = Only awakens when aroused
5 = Asleep at the time of charting

** Analgesic Rating Scale
(Please ask question verbatim)

Which of the following describes how you have felt over the last four hours?

1 = Comfortable
2 = In mild discomfort
3 = In pain
4 = In bad pain
5 = In very bad pain
AS = Asleep at time of charting

Appendix 1.7G: Drug Administration Record/Flowsheet

MEDICATION: _____ DATE: _____ CONCENTRATION: _____ mg/ml

Record hourly for first 4 hours after initiation or changes in dosing, then every 4 hours.				Record with each dose change.			Record every shift.		
Time	Respiratory Rate	Pain Rating	Sedation	Basal Rate mg/hr	PCA Dose mg	Lockout Delay min	Total CCs in new syringe after purging	CCs left at end of shaft	mg Infused per shift	signature

PAIN RELIEF SCALE

0 = No pain
1 = Uncomfortable
2 = Mild pain
3 = Distressing pain
4 = Moderate pain
5 = Severe pain

SEDATION SCALE

1 = Alert
2 = Drowsy
3 = Dozing intermittently
4 = Only awakens when aroused
5 = Asleep at observation

90

Appendix 1.7H: Drug Administration Record/Flowsheet

Epidural

Catheter Site _____

Drug-PF Morphine ☐ Fentanyl Infusion ☐ Other ☐ Specify _____

Postop Day	0	1	2	3	4	5	6	7	8	9
Narcotic Dose										
Injection Interval										
Pain (Rest)										
Pain (Move/Cough)										
Complications Resp Dep										
Itching										
N/V										
Urinary Retention										
Other										

Pain Scores: 0 - 10 (0 = no pain; 10 = worst possible)

Complications: 0 = none; 1 = mild; 2 = moderate; 3 = severe

Appendix 1.7I: Drug Administration Record/Flowsheet

Total Hours in Use	0	4	8	12	16	20	24	28	32	36	40	44	48
Date													
Time	am pm	am pm	am pm	am pm	am pm	am pm	am pm	am pm	am pm	am pm	am pm	am pm	am pm
Basal Infusion	mg	mg	mg	mg	mg	ml	ml	ml	ml	ml	ml	ml	ml
4-Hour Limit													
PCA Dose	mg	mg	mg	mg	mg	ml	ml	ml	ml	ml	ml	ml	ml
Lock-Out Interval													
Drug/Concentration													
Total No. of Doses Delivered	mg	mg	mg	mg	mg	ml	ml	ml	ml	ml	ml	ml	ml
Total Volume Dispensed													
Respiratory Rate													
Analgesia Level (see scale below													
Nurses Signature and Comments													

Document pain relief code in the comments column. Document in Nurses Notes every 8 hours
1 = pain free 2 = mild pain 3 = moderate pain 4 = severe pain

(For Pharmacy Use Only)

Filled Syringe

Total Volume Delivered

Volume Returned to Pharmacy and Wasted

Received and Wasted By _____

1st Witness Signature _____

2nd Witness Signature _____

Date received and Wasted _____

Appendix 1.8A: Acute Pain Service
Department of Anesthesiology
Physician's Orders for PCA

SUGGESTED DOSING REGIMENS

	Morphine Sulfate 1 mg/ml	Meperidine HCL 10 mg/ml	Hydromorphone HCL 0.2 mg/ml
PCA Dose:	1 to 3 ml (1mg-3mg)	1 to 2 ml (10mg-20mg)	1 to 2 ml (0.2mg-0.4mg)
Delay:	10 to 15 minutes	10 to 15 minutes	10 to 14 minutes
Basal Rate:	0 to 2 ml/hr (0-2mg)	0 to 2 ml/hr (0-20mg)	0 to 2 ml (0-0.4mg)
One Hour Limit:	4 to 7 ml (4mg-7mg)	4 to 7 ml (40mg-70mg)	4 to 7 ml (0.8mg-1.4mg)
Bolus Dose:	2 to 4 ml (2mg-4mg)	2 to 4 ml (20mg-40mg)	2 to 4 ml(0.4mg-0.8mg)

PCA INFUSION PUMP ORDERS   (Medication - please circle one)

Morphine 1 mg/ml		Meperidine 10 mg/ml		Hydromorphone 0.2 mg/ml

1. PCA DOSE   =   off   0.2   0.5   0.7   1.0   1.5   2.0   2.5   3.0   4.0   5.0   6.0   ML

2. DELAY   =   3   5   6   8   10   12   15   20   25   30   45   60   MINUTES

3. BASAL   =   off   0.5   1.0   1.5   2.0   2.5   3.0   4.0   5.0   7.0   8.0   9.9   ML/HOUR
   (Optional low dose infusion)

4. ONE HOUR LIMIT: = _____ ML

5. BOLUS: = _____ ML

6. If pain is not adequately controlled, select one of the following:

   a. Administer additional bolus doses of ____ ml every ____ hours - PRN may be given.

   b. PCA dose may be increased to _____ ml every _____ minutes PRN and the one hour limit increased to _____ ml.

   c. Increase basal rate to _____ ml per hour continuously and increase the one hour limit to ____ ml.

Date:	Time:	Physician Signature:

Appendix 1.8B: Acute Pain Service
Department of Anesthesiology
Physician's Orders for Intravenous PCA

DATE		**1**
TIME		

1. **Drug:** _____ MORPHINE (1 mg/ml)

_____ MEPERIDINE (10 mg/ml)

_____ OTHER _____ Concentration _____

2. Incremental Dose _____ mg, i.e., _____ ml.

3. Lockout Interval -- 8 minutes.

4. Four Hour Limit -- 30 ml.

5. If Pain not controlled after 1 hour, increase incremental dose to _____ mg, ie., _____ ml.

DATE		**2**
TIME		

6. If pain still not controlled after one additional hour, reduce lockout interval to _____ minutes.

7. No systemic narcotics or other CNS depressants to be given except as ordered by Acute Pain Service.

8. **Monitoring:**   Respiratory rate, analgesic level, sedation level - q2h for 8 hrs; then q4h. Record on ICU sheet.

9. **Documentation:**   Record drug use on ICU sheet at each monitoring interval and 8 hour totals on MAR.

10. **Treatment of Side Effects:**

DATE	A. DROPERIDOL 0.25 mg for severe nausea/vomiting. M R x 1 at 10 min. B. "In and out" bladder catheter prn for urinary retention.	
TIME	C. Call Acute Pain Service for sedation scale = 3. D. Call Acute Pain Service for RR < 8.	
	E. Give NALOXONE 0.1 mg IV STAT for sedation scale = 3 plus RR < 8. MR x 3. Call Acute Pain Service	**3**
	F. DIPHENHYDRAMINE 25 mg IV for severe itching. MR x1.	

11. For inadequate analgesia or other problems related to PCA, call Acute Pain Service.

Date _____   _____ , M.D.

Appendix 1.8C: Acute Pain Service
Department of Anesthesiology
Suggested Guidelines for Ordering PCA

ADDRESSOGRAPH

1. Analgesic via PCA infuser:
   Check one:

   Morphine 1 mg/ml
   Meperidine 10 mg/ml

2. Loading dose (optional, range 2-5 ml):
   If not administered in Recovery
   Room, give:
   Check one:

   Morphine 2 ml(2mg)
   Meperidine 2ml (20mg)
   _____ ml

3. Incremental dose (initial):
   Check one:

   Morphine 1 ml(1mg)
   Meperidine 1 ml(10mg)

4. Lockout interval (initial):

   10 minutes

5. Four hour limit:

   20 ml

6. If patient persistently complains of inadequate analgesia, check integrity of IV site.
   If IV is patent, increase dose volume to 1.5 ml (Morphine 1.5mg or Meperidine 15 mg).

7. If patient continues to complain of inadequate analgesia, check IV site.
   If IV is patent, decrease lockout interval to 8.0 minutes.

8. May repeat loading dose 2ml (Morphine 2 mg or Meperidine 20mg) q3-4 hrs.
   while sleeping and prn physical therapy.

9. Patient must have a running IV while PCA is in use.

   MD: _____

   DATE: _____

Appendix 1.8D: Acute Pain Service
Department of Anesthesiology
PCA Standing Orders

DATE & TIME		
	1. DISCONTINUE ALL NARCOTICS EXCEPT THOSE ORDERED BELOW.	
	2. ANESTHESIA PAIN SERVICE TO WRITE ALL NARCOTIC ORDERS.	
	3. _____ MG/ML TO BE DELIVERED BY A _____ PCA DEVICE.	
	4. P.C.A. VARIABLES:	
	- DOSE _____ MG (_____ ML)	
	- LOCKOUT _____ MINUTES	
	- _____ HOUR LIMIT _____	
	- CONTINUOUS BASAL RATE _____ ML/HR.	
	5. DROPERIDOL _____ ML (_____ MG) IV PRN FOR NAUSEA Q4H.	
	6. KEEP PCA PLUGGED TO WALL ELECTRICAL OUTLET EXCEPT FOR SHORT INTERVALS.	
	7. CHART RESPIRATION RATE Q4H ON PCA FLOW SHEET.	
	8. CALL PHYSICIAN FOR RESPIRATION RATE LESS THAN 10.	
	9. CHART PAIN LEVEL, LOC, AND PUPIL SIZE EVERY SHIFT ON PCA FLOW SHEET.	
	10. RECORD TOTAL _____ USED ON FLOW SHEET EVERY SHIFT.	
	11. NOTIFY APS FOR ANY PAIN PROBLEMS OR QUESTIONS ABOUT THE PCA.	
	12. IV: NS AT KVO IF NO IV ORDERS.	

Appendix 1.8E: Acute Pain Service
Department of Anesthesiology
Physician's Orders for Intravenous PCA

DATE	TIME	ORDERS	DOCTOR'S SIGNATURE	NURSE'S SIGNATURE
		DRUG AND CONCENTRATION: _____ _____ mg/ml.		
		LOADING DOSE: ___ NO ___ mg.		
		MODE: PCA _____, CONTINUOUS _____ ; PCA plus CONTINUOUS _____		
		PCA DOSE _____ mg		
		LOCKOUT INTERVAL _____ min.		
		CONTINUOUS RATE _____ mg/hour.		
		4-HOUR DOSE LIMIT _____ mg.		
		NOTIFY PAIN SERVICE PHYSICIAN BEFORE ADMINISTERING ANY SYSTEMIC NARCOTICS		
		PATIENTS MAY RECEIVE MEDICATION FOR SLEEP WHILE ON PCA (providing there is no continuous infusion)		
		Naloxone one ampule (Narcan 0.4 mg/ml) and Diphenhydramine (Benadryl 50 mg/ml) in patient's unit dose cassette.		
		If patient has nausea/vomiting:		
		yes ___ ; no ___ droperidol (Inapsine) 0.2 ml (0.5 mg) IV buretrol/push q2h prn x 2 doses.		
		IF NAUSEA AND VOMITING PERSISTS, CALL PAIN SERVICE FOR AN ALTERNATE TREATMENT.		
		yes ___ no ___ metoclopramide (Reglan) 20 mg IV buretrol (25-50 cc over 10-20 minutes)		
		q4h prn x 2 doses.		
		yes ___ ; no ___ transderm scopolamine patch over mastoid area while on PCA.		
		Monitoring - respiratory rate q2h x 8h; then q4h while on PCA. Please chart on daily record sheet with routine		
		vital signs.		
		Notify Acute Pain Service if the patient:		
		a) has a respiratory rate of 10 or less;		
		b) is difficult to arouse.		
		c) patient has an inadequate level of analgesia;		
		d) patient complains of pruritus (itching);		
		If there are any questions or problems related to PCA or if the pump alarms for malfunction, please call the Acute		
		Pain Service.		
		DATE _____ _____		_____ M.D.

Appendix 1.8F: Acute Pain Service
Department of Anesthesiology
Physician's Order Sheet for PCA Pump

EXECUTION			DATE/TIME	ORDERS	SIGNATURE/STATUS
Disposition	DATE	TIME	ORDERED		
				MEDICATION	
				LOADING DOSE ml	
				DOSE VOLUME ml (0.1-5.0)	
				LOCKOUT INTERVAL mins (5-99)	
				FOUR HOUR MAXIMUM ml (5-30)	
				NOTE MEDICATIONS AVAILABLE	
				MORPHINE SULFATE 1 mg/ml	
				MEPERIDINE 10 mg/ml	

Appendix 1.8G: Acute Pain Service
Department of Anesthesiology
Physician's Order Sheet for Continuous Epidural Narcotics

DATE	TIME	ORDERS	DOCTOR'S SIGNATURE	NURSE'S SIGNATURE
		Infusion: Drug(s) _____		
		Head of bed: _____ Activity: per surgeon.		
		VS per ICU routine; respiratory rate q1h; level of sedation q2hx4, then q4h.		
		Maintain IV access (drip or heplock) while epidural catheter is in place.		
		Pulse Oximeter. Please notify Acute Pain Service Physician if O2 saturation		
		is les than _____ %.		
		Naloxone (Narcan) 2 ampules (0.4mg/ml each) in patient's unit dose casette.		
		NO SYSTEMIC NARCOTICS TO BE GIVEN EXCEPT AS ORDERED BY ACUTE PAIN SERVICE.		
		Notify Acute Pain Service for:		
		a) increase of motor or sensory block.		
		b) somnolence or confusion		
		c) respiratory rate of 10 or less.		
		d) pruritus (itching)		
		For a respiratory rate of 10 or less, give Naloxone (Narcan) 0.1 mg IV push		
		(may be repeated every 5 minutes up to a total of 0.4 mg), and call the		
		Acute Pain Service STAT.		
		Treatment of Nausea/vomiting:		
		yes ___; no ___ droperidol (Inapsine) 0.2 ml (0.5mg) IV buretrol/push q2h prn x 2 doses.		
		yes ___; no ___ metoclopramide (Reglan) 20 mg IV buretrol q4h prn x 2 doses.		
		yes ___; no ___ transderm scopolamine patch over mastoid area for 24 hours.		
		Naloxone (Narcan) drip for prophylaxis of respiratory depression/itching:		
		yes ___; no ___ . Add ___ ampule(s) naloxone (Narcan 0.4 mg/ml)		
		___ per liter of maintenance IV fluid for ___ liter(s);		
		___ to 100 cc IV fluid (via buretrol) at ___ cc/hr x ____ hours.		
		If inadequate analgesia or any questions or problems related to Epidural, please call the Acute Pain Service.		
		DATE _____		M.D.

Appendix 1.8H: Acute Pain Service
Department of Anesthesiology
Physician's Order Sheet for
Post Surgical Continuous Epidural Morphine

EXECUTION			DATE/TIME	ORDERS	SIGNATURE/STATUS
Disposition	DATE	TIME	ORDERED		
				Duramorph 20 mg in 250cc NS. Run at _____ ml/h via pump	
				Begin at _____ (Range 5.0 - 12.0 ml/h)	
				Nalbuphine 40 mg in 500cc D51/2 NS. Run IV at 40 ml/h via pump	
				Begin at _____, run until complete.	
				HOB 30 degrees x 24 h if VS stable.	
				Check respiratory rate q1h x 18h.	
				Naloxone 0.4 mg in syringe with 9 ml NS at bedside. Give 0.04 mg (1ml) q1 minutes x 4 doses for respiratory rate less than 6/min.	
				For respiratory rate less than 6/minute, call APS stat.	
				Diphenhydramine 25-50 mg IM/IV hs prn sleep.	
				Droperidol 1.25 mg IV prn, N & V x 1 dose.	
				Nalbuphine 2.5 mg IV x 1 prn pruritus, N & V.	
				If pain is poorly controlled, call APS.	

Appendix 1.8I: Acute Pain Service
Department of Anesthesiology
Physician's Order Sheet for Continuous Epidural Opioids

EXECUTION			DATE/TIME	ORDERS	SIGNATURE/STATUS
Disposition	DATE	TIME	ORDERED		
				Sufentanil 200 mcg in 200 ml 0.125% bupivacaine. Run at _____ ml/h via pump. Begin at _____. If analgesia inadequate, increase rate to _____ ml/h (range 5.0-15.0 ml/h).	
				HOB 30 degrees x 24 h if VS stable.	
				Check respiratory rate q2h.	
				Naloxone 0.4 mg in syringe with 9 ml NS at bedside.	
				Give 0.04 mg(1ml) q1 minute x 4 doses for respiratory rate less than 6/minute.	
				For respiratory rate less than 6/minute, call APS stat.	
				Diphenhydramine 25-50 mg IM/IV hs prn sleep.	
				Nalbuphine 2.5 mg IV x 1 prn pruritus, N & V.	
				If pain is poorly controlled, call APS.	

Appendix 1.8J: Acute Pain Service
Department of Anesthesiology
Physician's Order Sheet for Post Surgical
Continuous Epidural Analgesia

DATE & TIME		ANESTHESIA Post-op Epidural Analgesia	TRANSCRIBED BY	OB-TAINED BY	CHECK POSTED OR CANCELLED	
					P	C
		(PLEASE CIRCLE ORDERS TO BE IMPLEMENTED AND COMPLETE BLANKS WHERE APPROPRIATE)				
		PACU: 1. Routine VS				
		2. Discharge from PAR per anesthesia care team				
		ON FLOOR: 1. On floor a) Apnea monitor _____ hours during bedrest, b) VS Q 4 , respiratory rate Q 1 , c) IMaintain patent IV, d) Tape 2 amps Narcan with syringe and needle @ bedside, e) Monitor for respiratory depression, f) If respiratory rate less than 8 per min., give 0.4 mg Narcan IV stat and and call anesthesia.				
		2. Epidural solution - circle one. Buretrol to be used. a) MSO 15 mg with Marcaine 150 mg in 150 cc NS, rate _____ cc/hr prn pain x 72 hr., b) Fentanyl 1500 microgram with Marcaine 150 mg in 150 cc NS, rate _____ cc/hr prn pain x 72 hr., c) Sufentanil 500 microgram with Marcaine 250 mg in 500 ccNS, rate 8-10 cc/hr/prn/pain.				
		3. Supplemental Medications a) MSO 2 mg IV, IM, or SQ Q2-4 prn pain, b) Emete-con 50 mg IM Q 4-6 prn nausea, c) Benadryl 25-50 mg PO, IV, or IM Q4-6 prn pruritus, d) If pruritus is unresponsive to 2 doses of Benadryl, give Narcan .080 mg IVP (dilute 1 amp Narcan with 4 cc NS in 5 cc syringe, give 1 cc of mixture. May repeat once Q 5 min.)				
		4. Nursing staff on floor call APS if any problems arise or catheter needs to be discontinued.				
		5. All other pre-op orders, medications, and diet per service with the exception of narcotics.				

Signed _____ M.D. Date _____

Appendix 1.8K: Acute Pain Service
Department of Anesthesiology
Physician's Order Sheet for
Post Surgical Single-dose Epidural Opioid

EXECUTION			DATE/TIME	ORDERS	SIGNATURE/STATUS
Disposition	DATE	TIME	ORDERED		
				HOB 30 degrees x 24 h if VS stable.	
				Respiratory rate q2h x 24h if stable.	
				Naloxone 0.4 mg in syringe with 9 ml NS at bedside.	
				Give 0.04 mg (1ml) x 4 doses for respiratory rate less than 6/min.	
				For respiratory rate less than 6/min. call APS STAT.	
				Diphenhydramine 25-50 mg IM/IV hs prn sleep.	
				Droperidol 1.25 mg IV prn N&V x 1 dose.	
				If pain is poorly controlled, call APS.	

Appendix 1.8L: Acute Pain Service
Department of Anesthesiology
Physician's Order Sheet for Post Surgical
Intermittent Intrathecal/Epidural Analgesia

DATE & TIME	DRUG ORDERS	
	1. Intrathecal/Epidural Duramorph ____ mg (dose) given at ____ (time), ____ (date).	
	2. Supplemental oxygen via nasal cannula @ 3 L/min. x 24 hours.	
	3. Vital signs q1 hour x 24 hours, then q4h.	
	Respiratory rate q30 minutes x 12 hours, then 1 hour x 12, then q4h.	
	4. Arterial blood gases q6 hours x 24 hours and prn respiratory distress.	
	5. Tape 2 amps of naloxone, 10 cc syringe, and 1 vial of normal saline dilute to the head o f the bed. If used for bolus, dilute 2 amps of naloxone with normal saline to 10 cc before administering.	
	6. If respiratory rate decreases to less than 8/minute x 3 minutes, give naloxone 80 mg IV push, and increase naloxone infusion by 0.5 mg/kg/hr.	
	7. Administer naloxone infusion (10 mcg/ml) via pump starting @ 1.0 mg/kg/hr. May increase the infusion by 0.5 mcg/kg/hr. increments over 3-5 minute intervals.	
	a) For pruritus, nausea or vomiting, may titrate as above but not exceed rate of 2.5 mcg/kg/hr.	
	b) For respiratory rate < 8/minute; or alterations of ABG's -- pH < 7.28, or pCO2 > 58, or pO2 < 65, may titrate as above bu not exceed rate of 4.0 mg/kg/hr.	
	8. Call M.D.:	
	a) if naloxone bolus given, or	
	b) if naloxone infusion rate reaches 3.0 mg/kg/hr., or	
	c) for uncontrolled pain, pruritus, nausea and vomiting, or continued respiratory depression.	
	9. For C/O pain, taper the naloxone infusion by increments of 0.25 mg/kg/hr q20 minutes until relief of pain, or to a minimum infusion of 0.5 mg/kg/hr.	
	10. Stop the naloxone infusion over 24 hours.	
	11. Do NOT give any parenteral narcotics x 24 hours.	
	12. After ____ (time) ____ (date) For further pain medication orders, call Anesthesia Pain Service.	
	13. For nausea and vomiting give droperidol 0.5cc (1.25 mg) IV, may repeat q4h.	
	14. If epidural catheter is still in place --	
	a) Observe the catheter insertion site for bleeding or leakage q2hrs.	
	b) Notify the APS if the catheter becomes dislodged and	
	c) No fluids or medications may be given via the epidural catheter.	
	15. Attach a sign/sticker "INTRATHECAL/EPIDURAL NARCOTICS" to the front of the patient's chart and the head of the patient's bed.	
	M.D.	

Appendix 1.8M: Acute Pain Service
Department of Anesthesiology
Physician's Order Sheet for Interpleural Catheters

DATE	TIME	ORDERS	DOCTOR'S SIGNATURE	NURSE'S SIGNATURE
		Drug: Bupivacaine:		
		a) Continuous infusion: concentration _____ ,		
		rate _____ cc/hr.		
		b) Bolus administration: concentration _____ ,		
		volume _____ cc.		
		Maintain IV access while interpleural catheter is in place. If surgeon has ordered an IV to be discontinued, please notify APS PRIOR to discontinuation, so that catheter can be removed.		
		NO SYSTEMIC OPIOIDS EXCEPT AS ORDERED BY ACUTE PAIN SERVICE.		
		For breakthrough pain, patient may receive:		
		yes _____; no _____ Nubain _____ mg every _____ hours prn		
		yes _____; no _____ Keterolac _____ mg every _____ hours prn		
		yes _____; no _____ Other: _____		
		Vital Signs:		
		a) CONTINUOUS INFUSIONS: per surgeon's routine.		
		b) INTERMITTENT BOLUSING: q15 minutes x 4 after each bolus administration. (APS resident will monitor		
		patient for first 2 sets of vital signs).		
		Notify APS resident for:		
		a) shortness of breath;		
		b) respiratory rate < 10, > 24;		
		c) bradycardia, HR < _____;		
		d) hypotension, B/P < _____;		
		e) change in mental status.		
		Chest x-ray within 1 hour after insertion of catheter and within 1 hour after removal.		
		Interpleural catheter is to be manipulated and/or removed ONLY by Acute Pain Service.		
		Notify Acute Pain Service in the event of:		
		a) inadequate analgesia		
		b) depletion of infusion		
		c) any problems or questions		
		DATE: _____ _____ M.D.		

Appendix 1.8N: Acute Pain Service
Department of Anesthesiology
Physician's Order Sheet for Pediatric Caudal/Epidural Analgesics

DATE	TIME	ORDERS	DOCTOR'S SIGNATURE	NURSE'S SIGNATURE
		DRUG: _____ DOSE: _____ ROUTE: _____		
		TIME ADMINISTERED: _____		
		NO OPIOIDS OR SEDATIVES FOR 12 HOURS AFTER ABOVE DOSE.		
		VS: At least q4h; respiratory rate q1h x 12h. Level of sedation q2h x 12h.		
		Do not discontinue working IV for 12 hours after above dose.		
		Naloxone (Narcan) ampules (0.4 mg/ml each) in patient's unit dose cassette.		
		Apnea monitor/pulse oximeter for 12 hours after above dose.		
		Notify Acute Pain Service in the event of:		
		a) excessive sedation (somnolence);		
		b) respiratory depression;		
		c) itching;		
		d) nausea/vomiting;		
		e) pain.		
		Any other questions or problems call the Acute Pain Service.		
		DATE: _____ M.D.		
		(Attending)		
		_____ M.D.		
		(Resident)		

Appendix 1.8O: Acute Pain Service
Department of Anesthesiology
Physician's Order Sheet for Pediatric PCA

DATE	TIME	ORDERS	DOCTOR'S SIGNATURE	NURSE'S SIGNATURE
		Drug and concentration _____ mg/ml		
		Mode: _____ PCA plus continuous infusion _____		
		PCA Dose: 0.02 mg/kg x _____ kg = _____ mg		
		Lockout Interval: _____ minutes		
		Continuous Rate (mg/hr):		
		0.02 mg/kg x _____ kg = _____ mg		
		4 Hour Limit:		
		0.02 mg/kg x _____ kg = _____ mg		
		VS: At least q4 hours; respiratory rate q2 hours x 8; then q4 hours.		
		Naloxone and diphenydramine in patient's unit dose cassette.		
		Notify APS in the event of:		
		a) inadequate analgesia		
		b) excessive sedation		
		c) respiratory depression		
		d) pruritus		
		If there are any problems or questions, please call the Acute Pain Service.		

Appendix 1.9: Drug Incompatibilities

Drug	Morphine	Meperidine
Amikacin	C	C
Ampicillin	C	C
Carbenicillin	C	C
Cefamandole	C	C
Cefazolin	C	C
Cefoperazone	C	I
Ceforanide	C	C
Cefotaxime	C	C
Cefoxitin	C	C
Ceftizoxime	C	C
Cefuroxime	C	C
Cephalothin	C	C
Cephapirin	C	C
Chloramphenicol	C	C
Clindamycin	C	C
Doxycycline	C	C
Erythromycin	C	C
Gentamicin	C	C
Kanamycin	C	C
Metronidazole	C	C
Mezlocillin	C	I
Minocycline	I	I
Moxalactam	C	C
Nafcillin	C	I
Oxacillin	C	C
Penicillin G	C	C
Piperacillin	C	C
Tetracycline	I	I
Ticarcillin	C	C
Tobramycin	C	C
Trimethoprim-sulfa	C	C
Vancomycin	C	C
Vibramycin	C	C

C = compatible

I = incompatible

Reprinted with permission from Compatibility of narcotic analgesic solutions with various antibiotics during simulated Y-site injection. *Am J Hosp Pharm* 1985;42:1108–1109.

Other incompatibilities
Morphine
Aminophylline
Amobarbital (Amytal)
Meperidine (Demerol)
Phenobarbital
Phenytoin (Dilantin)
Sodium bicarbonate
Thiopental sodium (Pentothal)
Zantac
Magnesium sulfate
Aminophylline
Diazepam (Valium)
Lasix
Hydrocortisone
Prednisone
Phenytoin (Dilantin)
Sodium bicarbonate

Naloxone is compatible with both morphine and meperidine.

If any question exists regarding the compatibility of an intravenous drug and the opioid being administered, Drug Information should be called.

PART II

The purpose of this section is to provide the basic concepts of newer pain modalities for acute pain management options in various patient populations.

6

Anatomy and Physiology of Pain

PHYSIOLOGY OF PAIN

The processing of nociceptive information is complex and is best considered by anatomical level. Peripheral nociceptors are specialized nerve endings that respond to different types of sensory input. Mechanoreceptors, including Meissner's corpuscles, Merkel's discs, and visceral corpuscles, respond to touch, pressure, and stretch. The impulses from these receptors are conveyed via A-delta fibers within the spinal nerve. Polymodal nociceptors are free nerve endings that respond to pressure, heat, and chemical irritation. Impulses from free nerve endings are conducted slowly via unmyelinated C-fibers. Nociceptive afferents release substance P and other algesic substances at synapses with second-order neurons in the dorsal horn of the spinal cord. In addition to peripheral nociceptors, pain receptors are also located in deep somatic structures, including skeletal muscle, joints, bones, and within abdominal and thoracic viscera. The afferent innervation of the viscera is via C-fibers traveling in the sympathetic nervous system. In the spinal cord, these afferents release substance P at the second-order neurons. Most nociceptive afferents terminate in the ipsilateral dorsal horn; some cross the midline and terminate in the contralateral dorsal horn. Others travel up or down within the spinal cord, synapsing at another spinal level. Rexed divided the spinal cord into 10 laminae; Laminae I–VI make up the dorsal horn; laminae VII–IX, the ventral horn; and lamina X is composed of those cells clustered around the central canal of the spinal cord. Lamina I of the dorsal horn is the marginal layer; lamina II comprises the substantia gelatinosa (SG), whereas laminae III–V is the region containing wide dynamic range (WDR) neurons.

Upon entering the spinal cord, the primary afferents take different courses depending on their size and function. C fibers tend to travel most laterally in the dorsal white matter, whereas the larger A fibers move more medially in the dorsal column. A delta fibers and their collaterals terminate at four sites: lamina I, lamina II, lamina V, and lamina X. C-fibers and their collaterals terminate in laminae I, II, and V. Afferents from muscle and other deep somatic structures terminate primarily in laminae I and V. Visceral afferents terminate predominantly in lamina I and V, but some also terminate in laminae IV, VI, VII, and X. The second order neurons then cross and ascend within the lateral spinothalamic tract contralaterally. The lateral or neospino-thalamic tract projects to neothalmus and the somatiosensory cortex, and mediates localization and discrimination of pain as well as noxious heat and cold sensation. The spinoreticular and paleospinothalamic tracts project to the brainstem reticular formation and limbic system, and mediate autonomic and motivational/affective responses to pain.

MODULATION OF PAIN

Modulation of Pain Occurs at Both the Spinal and Supraspinal Level

At the spinal level, nociceptive input is modulated by local release of endogenous opioids (enkephalin, dynorphin), which bind mu, kappa, and delta receptors at pre- and postsynaptic sites. Receptor activation inhibits further transmission of nociceptive impulses by limiting release of substance P or by stabilizing second order substantia gelatinosa cells. Brainstem control is primarily inhibitory and mediated by neurons of the periaque-ductal grey, reticular formation, and the nucleus raphe magnus. Descending adrenergic, enkephalinergic, and serotoninergic axons either inhibit primary nociceptive nerve endings or facilitate release of endogenous spinal opioids.

Higher Cortical (Psychological) Control

Emotional and cognitive mechanisms are able to modulate pain at various levels of the neuraxis and underlie individual variability in pain tolerance.

PSYCHOLOGY OF PAIN

The interaction of the psychological aspects of pain may add to the physi-ologic aspects of tissue injury thereby resulting in an exacerbation of the pain state. Many psychological factors, including fear, anxiety, separation, cultural and familial responses to pain, the patient's prior experiences with pain, as well as the surgical prognosis, influence the severity of postoperative pain. These are likely to contribute to a wide range of individual variations in response to a specific surgical procedure. The pain experience involves both the perception of sensory signal and the emotional reaction to that signal (1). In acute pain management, it is the behavior of the individual in pain that defines the severity of the pain problem for the hospital staff. The expression of pain is a behavior and is, therefore, shaped by learning. Social learning, or "learning by imitation," for pain-related behavior has cultural overtones. The context in which pain occurs will also influence pain behavior; uncertainty, loss of control, and social isolation will greatly influence the patient's expression of pain. Some of the methods of pain control discussed here minimize the uncertainty and return some control to the patient, hence improving the "pain state."

Much has been written on the psychology of pain, and we recommend referring to the texts listed as suggested reading for more detailed information.

PAIN ASSESSMENT

Pain assessment is a necessary step toward the satisfactory control of pain. Pain is assessed by observing the verbal and nonverbal behavior of the patient. Verbal behavior can, however, affect the accuracy of the assessment. Two "types" define the extremes of behavior in pain patients.

Stoic Patient

This person rarely complains of pain, which tends to be characteristic of at least one particular ethnic group. Members of the mainstream United States—particularly people who live in the Midwest or New England—often behave in a stoic fashion because they want to be thought of as "perfect patients." Asian-American patients may also behave in this manner (2).

Emotive Patient

This person is highly verbal regarding his/her pain, and can be problematic because too much data is forthcoming. Patients who vocalize discomfort and continually ask for relief are sometimes ignored. The reasons a patient may be emotive include fear, a desire for attention, grief, and the patient's cultural background (2).

Effective pain assessment must include education of the patient and staff: (a) Teach the patient to request pain medication or, if patient-controlled analgesia (PCA) is utilized, activate the device before pain increases to an unacceptable level of intensity. (b) Incorporate into the pain therapy that which the patient believes will be effective. (c) Consider the patient's ability or willingness to be active or passive in the application of pain control measures. (d) Institute and modify pain control measures on the basis of the patient's response. (e) If the pain control measure is ineffective the first time it is used, consider encouraging the patient to try it at least one or two more times before abandoning it. (f) A patient can be sedated and still in pain. (g) Anxiety and depression do not cause pain. They do make pain more difficult for the patient to tolerate and for the health care provider to manage. (h) When narcotics are withheld from patients who need them for pain relief, the result is clock-watching behavior. (i) Educate the patient regarding assessment scales. (j) Nonverbal behavior, such as grimacing or emotional withdrawal, communicate something whether or not the individual verbalizes it.

Numerous techniques for measuring pain have been used clinically to measure pain and its relief. Melzack (3) has written extensively on this topic, and the reader is referred to his work for an in-depth discussion of this topic. In acute pain management, healthcare providers rely on the patient to accurately assess pain. The Visual Analogue Scale (VAS) (4) provides a simple measure of pain intensity. The patient makes a mark on an unmarked line of 10 cm in length, anchored at one end with "no pain" and the other with "worst pain imaginable" (Fig. 6.1). This technique is easily understood by patients, and we use a VAS pain score of ≤3.5 to indicate adequate pain control. The VAS avoids the pitfalls of language involved in graphic rating scales, thereby avoiding individual interpretations to descriptors. There are, however, certain disadvantages to the VAS: (a) Some patients find it difficult to convert a subjective sensation to a straight line; b) teaching may not be adequate for accurate assessment; and c) VAS is an undimensional scale to measure intensity. However, the VAS, when used properly, is a reliable and valid pain measurement tool. Other methods of pain measurement and questionnaires include McGill Pain Questionnaire (Fig. 6.2), Numerical Rating (Fig. 6.3), Verbal Descriptor (Fig. 6.4), and the Faces Rating Scale (Fig. 6.5). The McGill Pain Questionnaire (3) has limited clinical use in acute pain management primarily due to its complexity and length, although it may be of great value in chronic pain management where it provides a qualitative assessment of pain.

REFERENCES

1. Beecher HK. Anxiety and pain. *JAMA* 1969;209:1080.
2. Greenwald HP. Intraethnic differences in pain perception. *Pain* 1991;44:157–163.
3. Melzack R. The McGill Pain Questionnaire: major properties and scoring methods. *Pain* 1975;1:275.
4. Gift AG. Visual Analogue scales: Measurement of subjective phenomena. *Nurs Res* 1989;38:286–288.

SUGGESTED READING

Wall PD, Melzack R. *Textbook of pain.* 2nd ed. New York: Churchill Livingstone, 1989.

MAKE A MARK ON THE LINE BELOW WHERE YOU FEEL YOUR

PAIN IS AT THIS TIME:

No Pain

Worst Imaginable Pain

FIG. 6.1. VAS Pain Scale.

Patient's Name _____ Date _____ Time_____am/pm

PRI: S_____ A _____ E _____ M_____ PRI(T) _____ PPI ____
    (1–10)   (11–15)   (16)   (17–20)   (1–20)

1 FLICKERING QUIVERING PULSING THROBBING BEATING POUNDING	11 TIRING EXHAUSTING
2 JUMPING FLASHING SHOOTING	12 SICKENING SUFFOCATING
3 PRICKING BORING DRILLING STABBING LANCINATING	13 FEARFUL FRIGHTFUL TERRIFYING
4 SHARP CUTTING LACERATING	14 PUNISHING GRUELLING CRUEL VICIOUS KILLING
5 PINCHING PRESSING GNAWING CRAMPING CRUSHING	15 WRETCHED BLINDING
6 TUGGING PULLING WRENCHING	16 ANNOYING TROUBLESOME MISERABLE INTENSE UNBEARABLE
7 HOT BURNING SCALDING SEARING	17 SPREADING RADIATING PENETRATING PIERCING
8 TINGLING ITCHY SMARTING STINGING	18 TIGHT NUMB DRAWING SQUEEZING TEARING
9 DULL SORE HURTING ACHING HEAVY	19 COOL COLD FREEZING
10 TENDER TAUT RASPING SPLITTING	20 NAGGING NAUSEATING AGONIZING DREADFUL TORTURING

BRIEF   MOMENTARY   TRANSIENT   RHYTHMIC PERIODIC INTERMITTENT   CONTINUOUS STEADY CONSTANT

E = EXTERNAL
I = INTERNAL

PPI
0 NO PAIN
1 MILD
2 DISCOMFORTING
3 DISTRESSING
4 HORRIBLE
5 EXCRUCIATING

COMMENTS:

FIG. 6.2. McGill Pain Questionnaire. Reprinted with permission from reference 3.

```
Instruction:  On a scale from 0 to 10, how strong is your pain?
0 = No pain 1  2  3  4  5  6  7  8  9  10 = The worst pain possible
```

FIG. 6.3. Numerical Rating Scale. Reprinted with permission from McGuire DB, Yarbro CH, *Cancer Pain Management*, Orlando, Grune & Stratton, Inc., 1987.

```
Instruction:  Which word best describes how your pain feels?


  None      Mild      Moderate      Severe      Excruciating
```

FIG. 6.4. Verbal Descriptor Scale. Reprinted with permission from McGuire DB, Yarbro CH, *Cancer Pain Management*, Orlando, Grune & Strutton, Inc., 1987.

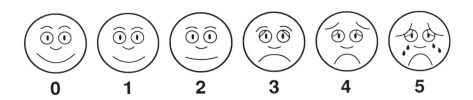

```
Face 0 = very happy, has no hurt.
Face 1 = still happy, but not quite as happy as "0".
Face 2 = isn't very happy or sad, is kind of "in between",
         hurts just a little bit.
Face 3 = sad, hurts a little more.
Face 4 = even more sad and hurts a whole lot.
Face 5 = is very, very sad; hurts as bad as can be.
```

FIG. 6.5. Faces Rating Scale. Reprinted with permission from McGuire DB, Yarbro CH, *Cancer Pain Management*, Orlando, Grune & Stratton, Inc., 1987.

7

Benefits of Analgesic Therapy

Ferne B. Sevarino, Raymond S. Sinatra, and Linda M. Preble

PAIN PREVENTION OR LACK OF PAIN PERCEPTION

This is achieved using spinal analgesia—with spinal opioids, local anesthetics, or a combination of two. (Fig. 7.1)

The advantages are that it (a) inhibits dorsal horn facilitation of pain transmission to higher cortical centers; (b) blunts sympathoadrenal response to pain (especially useful in patients with cardiac disease); (c) partially blunts neuroendocrine response (may decrease the release of stress hormones); and (d) greater preservation of preoperative pulmonary function.

The disadvantages are that it leads to (a) greater invasiveness; (b) greater risk of serious adverse events (i.e., respiratory depression, infection, neural trauma); (c) potential for hypotension, especially with local anesthetics; and (d) potential for urinary retention.

Risk/benefit ratio is highest in debilitated or high-risk patients recovering from large/painful procedures. Risks are minimized by utilizing continuous infusion techniques and continual monitoring in a high-visibility setting (e.g., Intensive Care Unit).

PAIN RELIEF

Pain relief is achieved with intravenous PCA, PCA plus a basal infusion and with regional blockade. (Fig. 1)

The advantages are (a) patient control—when compared with intramuscularly administered opioids, such therapy appears to increase patient satisfaction despite no apparent increase in the intensity of analgesia achieved;

$$\text{Overall patient satisfaction with therapy} = \frac{\text{Analgesic benefit}}{\text{Incidence and severity of side effects}}$$

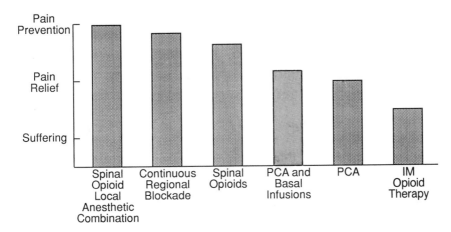

FIG. 7.1. Analgesic efficacy associated with various techniques.

(b) uniformity of analgesia—PCA overcomes a 4–5-fold interpatient variability in opioid dose requirement; and dosing is maintained by the patient, who is less dependent upon the health care provider. Eliminates the pain treatment cycle; and (c) titratability of analgesia—drug administration is titrated in relation to the intensity of the pain, i.e., PCA demands may be increased to overcome pain associated with movement/manipulation and decreased when interacting with visitors.

PCA-mediated "pain relief" is relatively safe and of greatest benefit to healthy low-risk patients recovering from moderately extensive/painful procedures.

8

Intravenous Patient-Controlled Analgesia

BACKGROUND

Patient-controlled analgesia (PCA) is a modality designed to accommodate the variable analgesic requirements that are seen in relation to postsurgical and other types of pain (1). PCA permits the patient to treat his/her own pain by direct activation of an infusion device that intermittently administers small doses of intravenous opioid. The rate of administration is controlled by the patient, within prescribed parameters, according to his/her own perception of pain. Individual drug titration provides for maintenance of an analgesic plasma concentration while avoiding either excessive or inadequate blood levels of opioid, thus reducing periods of excessive sedation or ineffective pain control (2) (Fig. 8.1).

The objectives of PCA are (a) to rapidly achieve effective analgesia with the smallest feasible dose of opioid; (b) to maintain continuous effective analgesia; and (c) to allow the patient to maintain a normal sleep pattern (3).

The small boluses and frequent dose intervals used with PCA, as opposed to intramuscular dosing given on an as needed basis (PRN), closely approximates a continuous infusion. Like continuous infusions, PCA has the advantage of minimal fluctuation in plasma drug concentration. Unlike continuous infusions, however, plasma levels with PCA do not depend to as great a degree on the constant elimination of the drug. PCA is titrated by the patient, and, thus, very stable, steady-state plasma levels are achieved as optimal analgesic concentrations are maintained. It is well recognized that with appropriate drug titration, opioid requirements may vary markedly among patients recovering from the same operative procedure (4,5). PCA permits the individual to titrate the opioid for the maintenance of analgesia, regardless of changes in either pharmacokinetic parameters, pharmacodynamic factors, or the varying intensity of the pain. Other advantages of PCA include (a) superior pain relief with less medication; (b) less sedation during

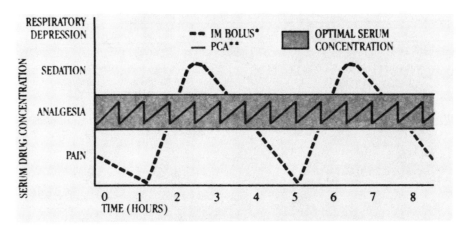

FIG. 8.1. IM dose-response compared to PCA dose-response objective. Reprinted with permission from Abbott Laboratories.

daytime hours; (c) improved respiratory function; (d) accommodation for diurnal changes; and (e) ability to titrate analgesic in response to need.

A major psychological advantage to PCA therapy relates to the ability to minimize the time delay between the perception of pain and the delivery of analgesic medication. For PCA to be successful the patient (a) should be given instructions preoperatively, for the operation of the PCA device; (b) should be informed that PCA use will not provide complete pain relief, but should make the pain tolerable; and (c) should be encouraged to use the device in a prophylactic manner to avoid the discomfort associated with ambulation, physical therapy, and dressing changes.

Extremely large doses of opioid may theoretically eliminate all pain. However, they cause unacceptable levels of respiratory depression and other side effects. An adequate level of analgesia, therefore, represents a compromise between tolerable pain and troublesome side effects. The patient should be encouraged to report any side effects that may occur so they may be appropriately treated. Table 8.1 outlines side effects and options for treatment. PCA pain management varies with each patient. Observation and assessment of the patient must be ongoing to determine individual therapy requirements, with adjustments being made when indicated. Tables 8.2 and 8.3 outline the means for objective assessment of pain relief and other side effects.

CLINICAL APPLICATION

Numerous PCA devices are currently available for use (see Appendix 2.2). The incorporation of a microprocessor into an infusion device permits activation of the pump by pressing a button connected to the apparatus. A

TABLE 8.1. *Treatment of side effects*

Condition/drug	Treatment
Pruritus	
Diphenhydramine 12.5–50 mg IV/IM	Be careful with increasing sedation, particularly in the elderly or debilitated patient under general anesthesia.
Naloxone 0.04 mg IV	May repeat after 5 min. May consider adding one ampule to a liter of IV fluid for 8–10 hr.
Nausea/vomiting	
Droperidol 0.25–0.625 mg	With larger doses, allow for the potential increase in sedation, secondary to potentiation of the narcotic. The weak alpha adrenergic effects of this drug may, with large doses, also cause hypotension.
Metoclopramide 20–50 mg IV	Increases gastric motility, has a central antiemetic effect, and less sedation than droperidol or compazine. Appears to be the antiemetic of choice for diabetic patients.
Transdermal scopolamine: one patch lasts 72 hr	In young, healthy patients (18–60 years old), this may be the antiemetic of choice. SCOP works well when patients complain of nausea with movement. A period of 4–6 hr may elapse before adequate levels are achieved. Another antiemetic must be used in the interim. In patients undergoing surgery with a high incidence of postoperative nausea. Consider placing a patch at induction of anesthesia.
Prochloroperazine—5–10 mg IM every 4–6 hr, 25 mg rectally every 12 hr	Will increase sedation May obscure intestinal obstructions May cause hypotension
Benzquimamide hydrochloride—IM 0.5–1 mg/kg to a maximum of 50 mg; IV 0.2–0.4 mg/kg to a maximum of 25 mg slowly	May cause drowsiness May cause hypo/hypertension
Trimethobenzamide hydrochloride PR 200 mg every 6–8 hr; PO 200 mg every 6–8 hr; IM 200 mg every 6–8 hr	IV or SQ administration is not recommended May cause extrapyramidal reactions Not as effective as phenothiazines in treating postoperative nausea
Promethazine hydrochloride—IM 25–50 mg every 4–6 hr; IV, PO, or PR 12.5–25 mg every 4–6 hr	May be given IV, IM, or added to the PCA syringe. SQ administration may cause tissue necrosis May cause sedation
Respiratory depression	
Stop PCA. Naloxone 0.04–0.1 mg IV (may be repeated in 5 min)	Leave PCA disconnected for a minimum of 1 hr. When restarted, decrease dose; discontinue basal rate if being used.

TABLE 8.2. *VAS pain scores.*

0 = No pain	1	2	3	4	5	6	7	8	9	10 = The worst pain possible

VAS pain scores of 2.5 to 3.5 on a 10-cm linear analogue scale (see Chapter 6) indicate adequate pain relief.

TABLE 8.3. *Observer sedation scores*

A five point scale provides useful documentation:
  1 = alert, oriented, initiates conversation
  2 = drowsy, oriented, initiates conversation
  3 = drowsy, oriented, *does not* initiate conversation
  4 = very drowsy, disoriented, *does not* initiate conversation—*closely observe, intervene as indicated!*
  5 = stupor, disoriented, *does not* initiate conversation—*intervention required!*

preprogrammed dose of opioid is administered over the 10–30-sec period following activation of the pump. With the administration of each opioid bolus, a lockout interval automatically begins thereby preventing the initiation of another dose during that time interval. Overdose is prevented by limiting the dose of opioid per bolus, the number of injections over a given time, and the total opioid dose over a given time interval.

Optimally, PCA is initiated postoperatively after the patient has been given a loading dose of opioid, either intraoperatively or in the postanesthesia care unit (PACU). The patient should be made analgesic prior to commencing PCA; otherwise, initial therapy will be complicated by the need to "catch up" with the pain. Patients using PCA usually use less opioid than the maximal amount available to them, and, if pain is adequately controlled, report Visual Analogue Pain Scores of 2.5–3.5 cm on a 10-cm scale. The following is a list of terms that one should be familiar with when ordering PCA:

Dose (increment): the amount of medication (in milligrams, micrograms, or milliliters) infused when the patient activates the control button

Basal rate (continuous infusion): the amount of medication per hour infused continuously by the device

Delay time (lockout): the time interval during which the patient cannot initiate a dose

4-hr (or 1-hr) limit: the maximum amount of medication the patient can receive during a 4-hr (1-hr) period. This governs the total amount of medication infused (basal and PCA doses combined).

Bolus (loading dose): the amount of medication (mg, μg, or ml) administered as either a loading dose or as additional doses to supplement PCA therapy.

Guidelines for PCA Therapy

1. PCA should not be offered to patients who would not normally receive parenteral opioids (i.e., those with an allergy to the prescribed opioid) or patients who are physically or mentally unable to operate the PCA pump.

2. For PCA therapy to be successful, healthcare personnel must understand the concept and the effects opioids have on the patient (Table 8.4).

3. The Acute Pain Service (APS) physician writes the prescription for PCA.

4. The APS physician should be notified before the administration of any other systemic opioids or sedatives while the patient is receiving PCA.

5. Although primarily offered to adult patients, patients as young as age 5 (see Chapter 11) may be deemed appropriate for PCA therapy.

6. The PCA infusion device should be locked at all times.

7. Treatment should be discontinued if, even after suitable adjustments in PCA therapy are made (ie. changes in drugs, dosages, or basal rate), a patient is dissatisfied with the therapy. Alternative pain medication should then be ordered by the patient's primary physician.

8. Standard postoperative monitoring is the minimum care for patients using PCA. Pulse oximetry and supplemental oxygen may be necessary for morbidly obese patients or other high-risk patients.

TABLE 8.4. *Effects of opioids on assessment parameters*

Parameter	Effect
Blood pressure	It must be remembered that hypertension may indicate hypercarbia secondary to overnarcotization. It must be remembered that opioids themselves usually do not cause hypotension. Hypovolemic states should be explored if hypotension occurs. Opioids, especially Morphine, can cause vasovagal reactions, which can cause hyper/hypotension.
Respiratory rate	8 *indicates significant narcotization and warrants a* discontinuation of a basal (continuous) infusion, decrease in PCA doses and possibly administration of a opioid antagonist.
Heart rate	May indicate inadequate analgesia (increase in heartrate) May indicate numerous postsurgical events (i.e. hyperthermia or a cardiac event).
Behavioral changes	Agitation—may indicate: Inadequate analgesia Hypoxia, possibly unrelated to opioid administration. Somnolence—may indicate: Overnarcotization Untoward postsurgical event Confusion—may indicate: Hypoxia Hypercarbia Untoward postsurgical complication (i.e. CVA or embolus)

VARIABLES AFFECTING THE EFFICACY OF PCA

All "components" of PCA may affect the efficacy of PCA therapy. These include the following.

Patient

Nature/Site of Surgery

Patients who have a large incision, (i.e., flank or thoracic) or who have undergone major orthopedic procedures have a greater need for pain medication than those who have had less extensive surgeries.

Psychodynamics

A "controlling" patient usually feels the need to have control during his/her hospitalization. PCA allows this patient to titrate opioids for acceptable pain relief. There are, however, some patients who can be classified "dependent" patients. (S)he prefers having a nurse administer analgesics, rather than controlling his/her own pain medication. PCA therapy will likely fail with this patient.

Psychotrauma

Good versus bad surgical outcome has an important psychological influence in pain management. Patients who have received less than optimal results from their surgery experience a greater amount of pain than a patient who had a more positive outcome. Thus, they have greater opioid requirements postoperatively.

Substance Abusers

Substance abusers are often demanding and manipulative. The use of PCA provided by a consult service eliminates pain therapy as a continual area of negotiation between patient and primary caregivers.

Age, Race, and Sex

Various authors suggest that these variables influence opioid requirements postoperatively (6,7) (see Chapter 11).

Adjuvant Drugs

Adjuvant drugs may influence opioid affects (see Chapter 10).

Disorders

Renal failure, liver failure, CNS disorders, and/or sepsis will influence the pharmacokinetics/pharmacodynamics of the opioid and thus the choice of opioid and the dose required.

Expectations

Kluger et al. (8) examined the expectations of patients using PCA (Table 8.5). His results emphasize that the patient's individuality should be maintained, that time spent with direct nursing contact should not be reduced, and that the machine should not replace the need for continual assessment by nursing staff. It is clear in his study that traditional nursing care and personnel contact are still of paramount importance to the patient regardless of pain management modalities utilized.

PCA Dose (Incremental Dose)

Generally, increasing the opioid dose leads to an increased incidence of side effects. Decreasing the dose may not provide adequate analgesia. Patients who are tolerant to opioids or who have had extensive abdominal or major orthopedic procedures usually require the greatest PCA bolus dose. The age of the patient is the most important variable in determining the PCA dose (6).

1. For healthy adults, a 50–70-kg adult can receive 1.0–1.5 mg of morphine every 6 min; or up to 2.0 mg every 10–12 min may also be utilized (0.2 mg/kg/hr divided into equal doses). Meperidine dosage in a 50-kg adult is 10–15 mg every 6 min; or 20 mg every 10–12 minutes may be utilized. With the larger doses, one sees an increase of side effects, especially nausea.

2. For elderly patients, 0.1 mg/kg/hr of morphine divided into 10 (every 6 min) equal doses may be adequate. Opioid clearance is decreased with age, and an increase in the clinical effect is seen.

3. In pediatric surgical procedures, morphine is the drug of choice for pediatric surgical procedures. The recommended dose is 0.05–0.1 mg/kg/hr. In a pediatric sickle cell crisis, morphine is the drug of choice for patients in vaso-occlusive crisis. The total dose of morphine is usually 0.1–0.2 mg/kg/hr. This is then divided into thirds, with two-thirds given as a continuous infusion and the remaining one-third divided into equal PCA doses.

TABLE 8.5. *Advantages and disadvantages of PCA (n = 74)*

Reason	Number
Advantages	
1. Not bothering nurses, nurses too busy with others.	30 (37.5%)
2. Rapid onset of pain relief	27 (33.8%)
3. In control of own pain relief	16 (20%)
4. Self-control, not losing autonomy	15 (18.8%)
5. Titrate exactly to needs	15 (18.8%)
6. Lack of injections	8 (10%)
7. No benefit	8 (10%)
8. Independence	5 (6.3%)
9. Reduction in the amount of pain	4 (5%)
10. Reassurance	4 (5%)
11. Not relying on nurses' assessment of pain	4 (5%)
12. Stable pain relief	3 (3.8%)
13. Helps research	3 (3.8%)
14. Mobilization better	2 (2.5%)
15. Will not worry other patients	2 (2.5%)
16. Reduction in amount of drugs	1 (1.3%)
17. Privacy	1 (1.3%)
18. Control of nausea	1 (1.3%)
Disadvantages	
1. No disadvantage	36 (45%)
2. Overdose	9 (11.3%)
3. Lack of nurse contact, less personal contact	9 (11.3%)
4. Over use, taking too much	8 (10%)
5. Machine dysfunction	5 (6.3%)
6. Inadequate analgesia	5 (6.3%)
7. Addiction	3 (3.8%)
8. Insecurity	2 (2.5%)
9. Over sedation	2 (2.5%)
10. No compassion	2 (2.5%)
11. Expense	1 (1.3%)
12. Restrict movement	1 (1.3%)
13. Needs intravenous cannula	1 (1.3%)

Reprinted with permission from ref. 8.

Phenergan (1–5 mg) may be added to the PCA syringe to enhance the analgesia and decrease the incidence of nausea and vomiting (see Chapter 11).

Lockout/Delay Time

Theoretically, the greater the time delay, the greater the margin of safety. However, a long lockout time may reduce patient satisfaction, as his/her ability to titrate analgesia in response to changes in the pain stimulus decreases. In addition, the ability to maintain adequate plasma levels is diminished. A shorter lockout interval is needed for rapid-onset, short-duration opioids, i.e., sufentanil, alfentanil, and fentanyl. A longer lockout interval is used for slower-onset, long-duration opioids, i.e., methadone.

Basal (Continuous) Infusion

The advantage of combining a basal infusion with PCA is to maintain minimum (subtherapeutic) plasma levels, allowing the patient to quickly achieve a therapeutic plasma level with PCA bolus doses (4). It improves ambulation by reducing movement associated pain and decreases pain intensity seen upon awakening.

The disadvantage of adding a continuous infusion is that it may decrease the intrinsic safety of PCA and may increase the likelihood of opioid tolerance. A high infusion rate may cause the blood plasma level to surpass the therapeutic threshold, and result in an increase in the incidence of somnolence and perhaps significant respiratory depression. This is especially true if patients are hypothermic ($\leq 36°$ C) immediately postoperatively and received large parenteral doses of intraoperative opioids.

A basal rate (Table 8.6 outlines guidelines) may be administered from the onset of PCA therapy if (a) this is protocol within your institution; (b) the performed surgery was extensive (i.e., a gynecologic-oncologic or major orthopedic surgery); (c) the patient is opioid tolerant as a result of long-term opioid use; (d) you anticipate inadequate pain relief with PCA alone; or (e) patient is in vaso-occlusive sickle cell crisis.

Loading Dose (Bolusing)

To achieve optimal benefit from PCA, the patient must be made comfortable prior to its initiation. A loading dose is necessary to obtain a baseline plasma level of opioid. This is accomplished by slowly titrating 0.05–0.1 mg/kg morphine (or the equivalent) either intraoperatively or in the PACU.

An additional loading dose may be necessary if the patient's IV infiltrates

---

TABLE 8.6. *Guidelines for adding continuous (basal) infusions with PCA*

Indications
    Extensive surgical procedures
    Opioid tolerance
    Inadequate analgesia with PCA alone
    Vaso-occlusive sickle cell crisis

Relative contraindications
    Age, >60 years
    Debilitated, malnourished patient
    Chronic lung disease
    Altered mental status

Monitoring considerations
    Pulse oximetry or apnea monitoring may be indicated

or the PCA syringe is exhausted, leaving the patient without opioid availability for a period of time. In these settings, plasma analgesic concentrations have become subtherapeutic and are best reestablished with bolus doses prior to restarting PCA. A loading dose may not be necessary if adequate doses of opioid were included in the intraoperative management or if PCA syringes are changed promptly. The PCA bolus dose is determined after the amount of opioid received intraoperatively, the amount received in the PACU and the degree of the patient's pain at the time.

With PCA, the administration of large bolus doses of opioid over a short time period will increase the incidence of side effects, particularly nausea and vomiting. Occasionally, a patient may experience dizziness or excessive sedation with large, frequent bolus doses. This rarely occurs with the administration of smaller bolus doses, given in 5–10-min intervals. Table 8.7 outlines guidelines for bolus doses.

Adjuvant Medications

The use of adjuvant medications while a patient is receiving PCA may enhance the effects of the opioid or may reduce opioid side effects. Appropriate adjustment should be made in the PCA dose increment and/or delay time (the dose may be decreased and/or the delay time increased) when indicated.

Adjuvants include the following:

1. Promethazine, 5–25 mg, may be added to the PCA syringe to decrease nausea/vomiting and pruritus. However, promethazine may potentiate the analgesic and sedative effects of the opioid.
2. Ketorolac, given every 6 hr, may decrease opioid requirements by one- to two-thirds. It is especially effective in patients recovering from orthopedic procedures.

TABLE 8.7. *Guidelines for bolus loading doses*

Every 5 minutes until the patient is comfortable, give:

Morphine, 1–2 mg, up to 30 mg
Meperidine, 10–20 mg, up to 100 mg
Oxymorphone, 0.1–0.25 mg, up to 1 mg
Fentanyl, 25–50 μg, up to 250 μg
Buprenorphine, 0.03–0.09 mg, up to 0.2 mg
Methadone, 0.5–3 mg, up to 15 mg
Dilaudid, 0.25–0.5 mg, up to 5 mg
Sufentanil, 2–10 μg, up to 50 μg
Nalbuphine, 1–5 mg, up to 20 mg

3. Metoclopramide (10–20 mg q 6 hr), administered IV, may reduce incidence/severity of nausea and vomiting. It also may potentiate analgesia, especially for patients who have visceral/colic pain.

4. Scopolamine, applied transdermally for nausea/vomiting prophylaxis or treatment, requires 4–6 hr to reach peak effect. One patch is active for 72 hr. It is not recommended for patients under 18 or over 60 years of age.

5. Benzodiazepines may be given to decrease muscle spasms, especially when associated with spinal surgery. They may also be patients with history of substance abuse.

6. Tricyclic antidepressants, used primarily for chronic pain syndromes, may "potentiate" the analgesic effects of opioids.

Analgesic

The ideal PCA drug for postoperative pain control would have a rapid onset, be highly efficacious, be of intermediate duration, have little abuse potential, and no adverse reactions. Unfortunately, this ideal opioid does not exist. There are, however, a large number of opioids that are available and can be utilized for PCA. Morphine and meperidine are the most commonly used. For the APS to be effective in meeting the needs of the individual patient, it should have the availability of a number of opioids to allow the choice of the most appropriate drug based on the nature/site of surgery and the patient's medical history. Table 8.8 lists available opioids and the dose ranges for PCA use.

The advantages and disadvantages of specific opioids are as follows:

1. **Morphine:** slow onset, long duration, significant histamine release, is best for somatic and orthopedic pain, less effective for visceral mediated pain; may increase visceral spasms/colic, may increase vagal tone, and may cause excessive sedation

2. **Meperidine:** rapid acting, moderate duration, less visceral spasticity in abdominal surgery than morphine, (especially procedures associated with significant visceral manipulation or ligation); has a lower incidence of nausea/vomiting, pruritus, and sedation than morphine

3. **Oxymorphone:** very rapid onset, prolonged duration, very high efficacy, less histamine release than morphine, but greater incidence of nausea/vomiting

4. **Hydromorphone:** rapid onset, moderate to long duration, high analgesic efficacy, lower incidence of histamine release than morphine; the incidence of sedation and nausea/vomiting are similar to meperidine, may cause confusion in elderly patients

5. **Fentanyl:** rapid onset, moderate duration, high incidence of sedation and nausea/vomiting; best as a continuous infusion in combination with PCA (continuous infusion plus PCA)

TABLE 8.8. *Intravenous PCA opioids*

Opioid	Adult	Adolescent
Morphine, 1 mg/ml or 5 mg/ml		
PCA dose	0.5–2.5 mg	0.5–2.0 mg
Delay	6–12 min	8–15 min
Basal	0–2 mg/hr	0–1 mg/hr
4-hr limit	Up to 35 mg	10–30 mg
Bolus	1–4 mg	0.5–3 mg
Meperidine, 10 mg/ml (one-tenth as potent as morphine)		
PCA dose	5–20 mg	5–20 mg
Delay	6–12 min	8–15 min
Basal	5–20 mg/hr	0–10 mg/hr
4-hr limit	Up to 300 mg	100–200 mg
Bolus	10–25 mg	5–15 mg
Oxymorphone (Numorphan), 0.1 mg/ml (6–10 times more potent than morphine)		
PCA dose	0.1–0.3 mg	
Delay	6–12 min	
Basal	0.1–0.2 mg/hr	
4-hr limit	Up to 12 mg	
Bolus	0.25–0.5 mg	
Hydromorphone (Dilaudid), 0.5 mg/ml (6–8 times more potent than morphine)		
PCA dose	0.1–0.5 mg	
Delay	5–15 min	
Basal	0–0.5 mg/hr	
4-hr limit	Up to 20 mg	
Bolus	0.25–0.5 μg	
Fentanyl		
PCA dose	15–75 μg	
Delay	3–10 min	
Basal	10–25 μg	
4-hr limit	0.3 mg	
Bolus	25–50 mcg	
Methadone[a]		
PCA dose	0.5–3 mg	
Delay	10–20 min	
Basal	Not recommended	
4-hr limit	Up to 50 mg	
Bolus	0–5 mg	
Buprenorphine (buprenex), 0.03 mg/ml		
PCA dose	0.03 mg	
Delay	8–12 min	
Basal	0–0.06 mg	
4-hr limit	Up to 0.8 mg	
Bolus	0.03–0.09 mg	
Sufentanil		
Dose	2–15 μg	
Delay	3–10 min	
Basal	1–3 μg/hr	
4-hr limit	160 μg	
Bolus	0–10 μg	
Nalbuphine		
Dose	1–5 mg	
Delay	5–15 min	
Basal	Not recommended	
4-hr limit	Up to 80 mg	
Bolus	1–5 mg	

[a]Use with caution as this drug has a 15-min onset and 12-hr half life, making the potential for significant respiratory depression greater than with other opioids.

6. **Sufentanil:** rapid onset, moderate to long duration; also best as a continuous infusion and PCA
7. **Alfentanil:** rapid onset, short duration may produce bradycardia; only effective as a combination of continuous infusion and PCA bolus doses
8. **Methadone:** moderate onset, long duration, long half-life, less sedation and euphoria than morphine
9. **Buprenorphine:** rapid onset, moderate duration; respiratory depression is not reversed with naloxone
10. **Nalbuphine:** rapid onset, moderate to long duration; has a respiratory depressant ceiling effect, but may increase sedation
11. **Butorphenol:** rapid onset, moderate to long duration; will increase systemic blood pressure and cardiac workload

Guidelines for the Use of Opioids for Specific Surgical Procedures

1. Patients recovering from major urologic procedures (i.e., suprapubic prostatectomies, cystocele repairs) and cholecystectomies usually do better with meperidine or hydromorphone than with morphine. Morphine appears to cause a high incidence of vasovagal reactions and increases complaints of spasmodic pain.

2. Gynecological patients, who have had tuboplasties and are on promethazine as part of an infertility protocol, do better with meperidine rather than morphine; morphine causes marked increases in sedation and an increase in respiratory depression.

3. Orthopedic patients achieve better levels of pain relief with morphine and dilaudid. Meperidine is less effective for periosteal pain. The PCA opioid is potentiated with the addition of a nonsteroidal antiinflammatory drug (i.e., ketorolac).

4. Oxymorphone, with a rapid onset and moderate duration, is an excellent opioid to "catch up" a patient who has inadequate pain relief. However, as a PCA opioid, it has a high incidence of nausea/vomiting and is very expensive.

5. Meperidine should be avoided in patients with a history of seizures. Its active metabolite, normeperidine, lowers the seizure threshold, and can precipitate seizure activity in susceptible patients.

6. The obstetric patient on magnesium sulfate for treatment of pregnancy induced hypertension is less sedated with meperidine than with morphine. However, as the seizure threshold in these patients is lowered, hydromorphone may be preferable.

7. Buprenorphine appears to be the drug of choice for renal transplant patients or in those patients who are at risk for significant respiratory compromise.

8. Hydromorphone, morphine, fentanyl and sufentanil are most potent, and therefore, should be considered as a first-line opioid choice in patients with extensive surgical procedures.

PROBLEMS WITH PCA THERAPY

Side Effects

Unacceptable side effects may be seen with large bolus doses and/or continuous infusions. Prompt recognition and treatment can do much to enhance PCA therapy and patient comfort and safety. Table 8.1 outlines the common side effects seen in patients receiving PCA and the usual therapies. The patient should be encouraged to report any side effects to allow prompt treatment and, thus, optimal benefit of the therapeutic regimen.

Problems with the PCA Infusion Device

The following are problems that can occur with the PCA infusion device (9):

1. Operator errors
   a. Misprogramming PCA device
   b. Failure to clamp or unclamp tubing
   c. Improperly loading syringe or cartridge
   d. Inability to respond to safety alarms
   e. Misplacing PCA pump key
2. Patient errors
   a. Failure to understand PCA therapy
   b. Misunderstanding PCA pump device
   c. Intentional analgesic abuse
3. Mechanical errors
   a. Failure to deliver on demand
   b. Defective one-way valve at Y connector
   c. Faulty alarm system
   d. Malfunctions (e.g., software)

SUMMARY

PCA is a system designed to accommodate the wide range of analgesic requirements that can be anticipated when managing acute postoperative pain. In the postoperative setting, PCA is utilized for the maintenance of analgesia; the patient should be analgesic prior to initiation. If PCA is to be successful, the bedside nurse should be skilled in the assessment of pain so that the individual patient's response to therapy can be monitored effectively (10). Inadequate analgesia, overnarcotization, or side effects that persist must be reported to the APS so that the optimum benefit of PCA can be achieved.

REFERENCES

1. Ferrante MF, Ostheimer GW, Covino BG. *Patient controlled analgesia.* Cambridge MA: Blackwell Scientific Publications, 1990.
2. White PF. Use of patient-controlled analgesia for management of acute pain. *JAMA* 1988; 259:243–247.
3. White PF. Patient-controlled analgesia: a new approach to the management of postoperative pain. *Semin Anesthiol* 1985;4:255–266.
4. Owen H, Szekely SM, Plummer JL, Cushnie JM, Mather LE. Variables of patient-controlled analgesia 2. concurrent infusion. *Anaesthesia* 1989;44:11–13.
5. Burns JW, Hodsman NBA, McLintock TTC, Gillies GWA, Kenny GNC, McArdle CS. The influence of patient characteristics on the requirements for postoperative analgesia. *Anaesthesia* 1989;44:2–6.
6. Owen H, Kluger MT, Plummer JL. Variables of patient-controlled analgesia 4: the relevance of bolus dose size to supplement a background infusion. *Anaesthesia* 1990;45: 619–622.
7. Bellville JW, Forrest WH, Miller E, Brown BW. Influence of age on pain relief from analgesics. JAMA, 1971;217:1835–1841.
8. Kluger MT, Owen H. Patients' expectations of patient-controlled analgesia. *Anaesthesia* 1990;46:1072–1073.
9. White PF. Mishaps with patient-controlled analgesia (PCA). *Anesthesiology* 1987;66: 81–83.
10. Atsberger DB, Shrewsbury P. Postoperative pain management: the PACU nurse's challenge. *J Post Anesthesia Nursing* 1988;3:399–403.

SUGGESTED READING

White PF. Patient-controlled analgesia. *Problems in Anesthesia* 1988;2:339–350.
Benzon HT. Postoperative pain and its management. *Resident and Staff Physician* 1989;35: 21–26.
Tamsen A, Hartvig P, Fagerlund C, et al. Patient-controlled analgesic therapy—clinical experience. *Acta Anaesthiol Scand* 1982;74:157–160.
Weis OF, Sriwatanakul K, Allozo JL, et al. Attitudes of patients, housestaff, and nurses toward postoperative analgesic care. *Anesth Analg* 1983;62:70–74.

9

Spinal Opioids

Raymond S. Sinatra and Ferne B. Sevarino

The high quality and superior effectiveness of analgesia provided by intraspinal opioids have clearly advanced the management of postsurgical, obstetrical, and chronic pain. In the brief span of 10 years, numerous articles and citations have confirmed the efficacy of intraspinal administration of opioids and their ability to provide analgesia without associated motor blockade or excessive central nervous system (1,2) depression. Proper use of intraspinal opioids allows for early ambulation, as well as improved pulmonary function with increased ability to cough and clear respiratory secretions, and greater patient comfort than traditional methods of pain relief (3–5).

BACKGROUND

It has been shown that specific opioid receptor binding in the substantia gelatinosa (lamina I and II) provides analgesia; nociceptive input is effectively blunted at the first synapse in the CNS. Evidence supporting spinal opioid activity includes (a) neurophysiological studies demonstrating selective suppression of nociceptive neurons following spinal administration of morphine (6); (b) studies demonstrating significant reductions in dorsal horn opioid binding following rhizotomy (7); and (c) behavioral studies demonstrating that small doses of intrathecal morphine produce prolonged analgesia that can be reversed by naloxone (8,9).

To understand the benefits as well as the complications of spinal opioid analgesia one must appreciate the pharmacokinetics of the agents used. Opioids administered intrathecally or epidurally provide selective analgesia which occurs with an absence of motor or sympathetic blockade. Epidural administration is complicated by factors related to dural penetration, absorption into fatty tissue and systemic uptake. Spinal administration of opioids produces dose-dependent analgesia of greater potency than similar doses administered parenterally. This greater potency is inversely related to lipid solubility. Although many factors affect analgesia, including dose, volume of injectate, and molecular weight and shape, the factor with the greatest influence on the onset, dermatomal spread, and duration of analgesia appears to be lipid solubility. In this regard, the delayed analgesic onset noted with epidural administration of morphine is related to its low lipid solubility which reduces dural permeability and thus retards the penetration into spinal tissue. Following administration, significant amounts of drug are sequestered in the CSF. This aqueous "depot" of unbound morphine allows for a prolonged duration of analgesia, but is the underlying cause of delayed respiratory depression (10,11).

Recognition that delayed respiratory depression and other side effects can be attributed to the retention and rostral spread of hydrophilic morphine molecules has led investigators to examine lipid soluble agents. These agents leave the CSF and rapidly bind to lipid rich spinal tissue and thus do not spread rostrally in the CSF. Commonly utilized lipophilic agents include the phenylpiperidine derivatives meperidine, fentanyl, and sufentanil. In general, lipophilic opioids provide a more rapid onset of analgesia than does morphine but a shorter duration. Although these agents are not associated with a high incidence of pruritus or delayed respiratory depression, "early onset" respiratory depression has been observed. This usually occurs within 30 min of administration and is related to intravenous uptake of the opioid.

CLINICAL APPLICATION

The pharmacodynamics and pharmacokinetics of intraspinal opioids are important in determining the dosage and the extent of dermatomal spread. The benefits of spinal opioids, as mentioned above, include excellent analgesia, better postoperative pulmonary function, earlier ambulation, and a decrease in morbidity and mortality (3,4). The goal is to use the lowest effective dose that will ensure adequate analgesia, and yet minimize opioid-related side effects.

Guidelines for Clinical Use of Intraspinal Opioids

1. All patients receiving spinal opioid analgesia must have either a patent intravenous or heparin lock in place.
2. The anesthesiologist will determine which, if any, patient(s) require apnea monitoring or pulse oximetry. The following patients are at higher risk for respiratory depression:
   a. Those who are ≥50 years of age
   b. Those with moderate to severe systemic disease that produces functional limitation (ASA physical status of >II)

   c. Those who have received large doses of spinal opioids (e.g., ≥ 5 mg epidural morphine or ≥ 1 mg subarachnoid morphine)

   d. Those who have undergone prolonged surgery

   e. Those who had opioids administered at a thoracic site (via thoracic epidural catheter)

3. The epidural (or subarachnoid) catheter must be clearly identified and labeled to prevent accidental administration of solutions/medications intended for intravenous use.

4. The use of a transparent dressing, (e.g., TEGADERM), to cover the catheter at the insertion site will facilitate assessment of the site. The catheter will be taped securely to the back. With intermittent bolus administration, the injection port should be capped between doses to ensure sterility.

5. AT NO TIME IS ANY MEDICATION TO BE ADMINISTERED THROUGH THE INJECTION PORT OTHER THAN THE OPIOID OR OPIOID/LOCAL ANESTHETIC MIXTURE. THIS IS TO BE DONE ONLY BY THE ANESTHESIOLOGIST OR BY A PROFESSIONAL UNDER HIS/HER DIRECT ORDER.

6. The patient is to be assessed daily by the Acute Pain Service (APS) team and a note made in the history and progress notes or on follow-up progress notes. Assessment includes level of pain relief, appearance of catheter insertion site, side effects, and requisite treatments.

7. Nursing personnel shall monitor the patient frequently.

   a. Level of sedation and respiratory rate should be checked every hour and charted by the nursing staff for the entire duration of a continuous infusion, and for 8 hr following administration of a single dose of spinal morphine, then every 2 hr for the next 16 hr.

   b. Level of sedation

      i. None: alert

     ii. Mild: occasionally drowsy; easy to arouse

    iii. Moderate: frequently drowsy; easy to arouse

    iv. Severe: somnolent; difficult to arouse; patient disoriented/confused

8. An epidural catheter may be kept in place for up to 7 days; subarachnoid catheters for 2 days, providing the patient's temperature remains $< 101°F$ ($39°C$). If the patient becomes febrile (temperature of $> 101.5°F$, $39.5°C$) on or after the third day of therapy with an epidural catheter, or at any time with a subarachnoid catheter, the insertion site should be examined for signs of infection. If there is purulent drainage, the catheter should be removed and sent for culture and sensitivity. In the initial postoperative period (1–2 days postoperatively), temperature spikes are common and are usually secondary to atelectasis; therapy may continue if the patient is clinically stable and there is no evidence of sepsis.

9. Management of patients with catheters who are receiving anticoagulants
   a. In patients started on warfarin (Coumadin) following catheter insertion, catheters may remain in place.
   b. Catheters may remain in place in patients receiving intermittent heparin (usually subcutaneous) therapy.
   c. In patients who will be receiving a continuous heparin infusion, catheter removal is controversial. Some clinicians believe that if a heparin infusion has been started with the catheter not yet removed, the patient's prothrombin time and partial thromboplastin time (PT/PTT) should be checked, and if these are within normal limits, the catheter should then be discontinued immediately. If the PT/PTT are elevated, the infusion should be discontinued to allow for removal of the catheter when the PT/PTT normalize. If it is not possible to temporarily discontinue the heparin, the catheter should be left in place (but not used for analgesia) until coagulation parameters can be returned to normal (i.e., heparin discontinued) and it can safely be removed. In all cases, the patient must be monitored for signs of severe back pain and/or muscle weakness which would indicate an epidural hematoma. Other clinicians believe spinal opioid analgesia is safe and not associated with epidural hematomas in patients who are heparinized and would thus maintain spinal analgesia in these patients.
10. Leaking catheters
   a. For catheters that are leaking but not disconnected from the connector site, the connector should be changed. This usually corrects the problem.
   b. Catheters disconnected from the connector and thus contaminated should be discontinued.
   c. Catheters leaking at the insertion site should be evaluated by the anesthesiologist.

Discontinuation of Therapy

1. The decision to stop an infusion is based on several factors
   a. Migration of the catheter from the epidural or subarachnoid space
   b. The patient's status
   c. In institutions where this therapy is not permitted on the patient care unit, the transfer of the patient from an intensive care unit to a patient care unit.
2. There are several methods for discontinuing an infusion
   a. The infusion is stopped.

b. If the infusion contains local anesthetics, the local is deleted from the solution and a pure opioid is infused for several hours prior to discontinuing the infusion.

c. The patient is weaned slowly (ie. the rate of infusion gradually decreased), irregardless of solution mixture (i.e. opioid and local anesthetic).

d. The patient is given an intramuscular opioid injection and the infusion stopped 30 min later.

e. The patient is given an oral opioid and infusion is discontinued 2 hr later. Patients with cerebrovascular or heart disease (coronary artery, valvular and cardiomyopathy) should be weaned gradually from the infusion if it contains local anesthetics in concentrations greater than 0.05%. Pulmonary edema followed by a cerebrovascular accident (CVA) or myocardial infarction can occur following abrupt discontinuation of epidural analgesia. This may be secondary to the sudden loss of sympathetic blockade, with a resulting central volume overload. Thus, for this patient population, we recommend the rate of infusion be decreased by 50% for 4–8 hr and then stopped, or that it be decreased slowly by 2 ml every 2 hr.

Variables

Opioid

Morphine

Epidural Administration. Epidural morphine (preservative free: Duramorph, Astramorph) is administered at lumbar sites in doses ranging from 3 to 10 mg in diluent volumes of 10–20 ml (12) (Table 9.1). Epidural morphine requirements for patients recovering from gynecological surgery appear to be inversely related to patient age, with the 24-hr dose requirement in milligrams equivalent to $(18 - age) \times (0.15)$ (13). Thoracic sites of administration $(T_{12} - T_6)$ are recommended for control of upper abdominal or thoracic pain. With thoracic administration, the morphine dose is reduced by one-third to one-half, and the diluent volume halved as well.

Continuous epidural infusions of morphine or bupivacaine/morphine in combination are highly effective in controlling the severe pain associated with upper abdominal and thoracic surgery. Continuous infusions (morphine, 0.5–1.0 mg/hr) provide excellent analgesia, without the systemic side effects observed with intermittent epidural dosing (14). Morphine dose requirements are influenced by patient age, height, location of administration, and the site and extent of surgery. The usual epidural dose is 5 mg in 10 ml volume given through a lumbar catheter for incisions below T_{10}. This provides adequate analgesia of a long duration (18–24 hr) with minimal side

TABLE 9.1. Recommended doses of interspinal opioids

Drug	Epidural dose	Peak effect (min)	Duration (hr)	Intrathecal dose	Peak (min)	Duration (hr)
Morphine	3–10 mg	90–120	8–24	0.1–0.5 mg	15–30	8–24
Fentanyl	50–100 µg	10–15	2–4	6.25–15 µg	5–10	4–6
Sufentanil	25–50 µg	10	3–5	2.0–7.5 µg	5–10	3–5
Meperidine[a]	25–50 mg	15 min	4–6	10 mg	15	4–6
Methadone	3–10 mg	10–30	6–8	2 mg	15	4–6
Morphine and fentanyl	3–5 mg Morphine/50 µg fentanyl	10 min	8–24			
Morphine and sufentanil	3–5 mg Morphine/30 µg sufentanil	10 min	6–24			

[a]Meperidine is usually used in a continuous infusion in combination with low-dose bupivacaine.
Doses should be decreased for older patients: by 20% for those over 60 years, by 40% for those over 70, and by 60% for those over 80.

effects. The slow onset (30–60 min with 90–120 min to peak effect) requires that morphine be given at least 1 hr before the patient awakens from general anesthesia, before regression of an epidural anesthetic, or in combination with a more rapidly acting, lipophilic opioid (e.g., fentanyl, sufentanil).

Morphine and fentanyl in combination provide a more rapid onset and a slightly shorter duration than morphine alone. The usual bolus dose is 50 μg fentanyl and 3–5 mg of morphine in a total volume of 10 ml. With this combination, onset is in 15 min and duration is 8–20 hr. For patients over 60, decrease the dose by 20%; over 70, 40%; over 80, 60%; and over 90, 80%.

Intrathecal Administration. Intrathecally administered morphine has been shown to improve postoperative analgesia and pulmonary function, especially in patients recovering from orthopedic, gynecological, and genitourinary surgery (3–5). Intrathecal morphine has also been useful in gallbladder surgery; doses of 0.2 mg provided up to 24 hr of complete analgesia with a minimal risk of precipitating sphincter of Oddi spasm (15). With the development of 28- and 32-gauge catheters, continuous administration of intrathecal morphine offers the advantage of potent, highly selective analgesia along with improved versatility in dosing (16).

Monitoring. Following spinal administration of morphine, or after the initiation of a continuous infusion, all patients over age 60 and/or with moderate to severe systemic disease (e.g., insulin dependent diabetes mellitus, chronic obstructive lung disease) should be admitted to an intensive care unit for 16–20 hr.

Fentanyl

Epidural Administration. Fentanyl is the lipophilic opioid of choice for epidural analgesia. Its highly efficacious, safe, and is commonly employed to control postoperative and obstetrical pain. It is often difficult to achieve rostral spread of fentanyl, as it is rapidly cleared from epidural and spinal sites of deposition. This explains its "segmental" analgesic properties. With lipophilic agents, the rate of dural penetration and dermatomal spread appears to be directly related to the surface area which comes in contact with the drug. Thus, fentanyl may be more effective in blunting pain associated with upper abdominal and thoracic surgery when administered either in larger diluent volumes or by continuous infusion.

Epidural fentanyl may be combined with subtherapeutic doses of bupivacaine to achieve "supra-additive" postsurgical analgesia. This technique is especially useful in patients who have pulmonary or cardiac disease and cannot tolerate intercostal muscle weakness or the sympathectomy associated with greater concentrations of local anesthetic. For postoperative analgesia following upper abdominal thoracic surgery, we recommend a continuous infusion of fentanyl via a thoracic epidural catheter. Placing the catheter immediately adjacent to opioid receptors in the thoracic region of the spinal cord reduces the total fentanyl dose by 50% and will thus minimize systemic uptake and central effects.

Intrathecal Administration. Fentanyl 6.25 μg or 12.5 μg given in combination with bupivacaine 0.75% improves perioperative anesthesia, but provides little if any postoperative analgesia. Intrathecal use of fentanyl for postoperative analgesia would only be effective with repeated boluses through an indwelling catheter or as a continuous infusion.

Meperidine

Epidural Administration. The physicochemical properties of meperidine, which include a moderately high lipid solubility, mu receptor specificity, and local anesthetic properties, make it useful in this setting. In recent years, meperidine has been used increasingly as an agent for continuous epidural infusion. Its lipophilic characteristics are intermediate between morphine and fentanyl, and are similar to those of bupivacaine; with epidural infusions of 0.1% meperidine and 0.1% bupivacaine in combination, both agents appear to spread equally and to provide synergistic analgesic benefit (18,19).

Intrathecal Administration. Intrathecal meperidine 5–20 mg in combination with bupivacaine 0.75% provides excellent perioperative anesthesia and postoperative analgesia of approximately 4–6 hr in duration.

Sufentanil

Epidural Administration. Sufentanil is currently in the final phase of FDA evaluation. Approval for use as an epidural analgesic is expected soon. The key findings of a number of clinical studies all indicate that sufentanil provides extremely rapid and effective postoperative analgesia with no evidence of delayed respiratory depression. However, dose requirements are high, early-onset ventilatory depression occurs, and the duration of pain relief, although dose dependent, is apparently no greater than that provided by fentanyl (18,20).

Sufentanil is most effective when administered by continuous epidural infusion. This method takes advantage of the agent's rapid onset and short duration, and minimizes the respiratory risks associated with large bolus doses. For patients recovering from intraabdominal surgery, lumbar infusions of 0.3 μg/kg/hr provided rapid and sustained analgesia with minimal side effects (21). Greater selectivity and reduced dose requirement (0.1–0.2 μg/kg/hr) have been seen when sufentanil is administered through thoracic catheters.

Intrathecal Administration. Small doses (5 μg) of intrathecal sufentanil can produce approximately 3–5 hr of analgesia (22).

Other Agents

Other lipophilic opioids include hydromorphone, heroin, methadone, butorphanol, and buprenorphine. These also reportedly provide effective analgesia following epidural administration (23,24). However, none provide any advantage over the more commonly used opioids. Although the onset of analgesia is more rapid with epidural methadone (5 mg) and hydromorphone (1 mg) than with morphine (5 mg), the duration is not as long (7 and 11 hr, respectively). It is not clear if the risk of "delayed" onset respiratory depression or other adverse effects is lower with hydromorphone than with morphine. However, a preservative free preparation is now commercially available for epidural administration.

Both the lipophilic mixed-agonist butorphanol (23) and the partial agonist buprenorphine have limited utility because as significant central effects result from systemic absorption and recirculation to the CNS. In this regard, epidural butorphanol produces a dose dependent increases in sedation and parallel increases in analgesic duration. Buprenorphine also produces dose dependent increases in sedation, which may be difficult to reverse, even with high doses of naloxone.

Lipophilic opioids are less commonly administered intrathecally. The limited duration of analgesia provided usually does not warrant the potential risk of dural puncture, headache, infection and neurotoxicity. At present, these are most frequently used as adjuncts to spinal anesthesia.

Mode of Administration

Intermittent Bolus Administration

Intermittent epidural bolus administration is best with opioids of with long duration, primarily morphine. Shorter duration opioids (i.e., lipophilic) provide better analgesia if utilized as continuous infusions, either epidural or intrathecal. Bolus doses of intrathecal opioids, may provide superior intraoperative anesthesia in combination with local anesthetics. Morphine, meperidine, and sufentanil provide analgesia of sufficient duration to warrant a single dose or intermittent bolus injection for postoperative analgesia.

Continuous Infusion Drugs

Use of continuous epidural infusions provides long-lasting uniform analgesia, whereas at the same time decreasing the severity and/or incidence of side effects as compared to intermittent bolus administration. They do not cause the high peak CSF levels that accompany intermittent bolus administration (Table 9.2).

Morphine. This (Astramorph and Duramorph) is used for large incisions that require a wide dermatomal distribution of analgesia. There is risk of migration of this agent in the CSF to the brainstem, causing respiratory depression. When used in combination with dilute concentrations of bupivacaine, morphine dose requirements are greatly decreased and therefore, morphine related side effects and are decreased as well.

Fentanyl. This is highly lipid soluble, thus does not migrate cephalad in the CSF. With large doses, significant uptake by the epidural vasculature occurs, resulting in high systemic concentrations which may lead to sedation and respiratory depression. As with morphine, lower doses may be used if combined with dilute bupivacaine.

Meperidine. This is most effective when used as a continuous infusion and when used in combination with dilute local anesthetic solutions. It is 20 times more lipid soluble than morphine, and thus has less tendency to migrate cephalad. As a result, delayed respiratory depressions does not occur. Meperidine is moderately lipophilic, but is not taken up systemically in significant amounts.

Hydromorphone. This has a faster onset, but a shorter duration of action than dose epidural morphine. A certain amount of rostral spread probably occurs in the CSF with hydromorphone, thereby creating the potential for delayed respiratory depression.

Sufentanil. This has a very rapid onset without the possibility for delayed respiratory depression. In bolus doses, sufentanil provides no greater duration of pain relief than does fentanyl and thus continuous infusions should be utilized. (25)

Use of Local Anesthetics With or Without Opioids

Local anesthetics, injected epidurally in relatively high concentrations and large volumes, provide surgical anesthesia. Smaller doses injected into the subarachnoid space have the same effect. This results in afferent and

TABLE 9.2. *Epidural infusions*

Combination therapy Bupivacaine	and	Fentanyl	or	Morphine	or	Meperidine
0.02–0.25% (0.2–2.5 mg/ml)		0.0005–0.001% (5–10 µg/ml)		0.005–0.01% (0.05–0.1 mg/ml)		0.1% (1 mg/ml)

Infusion rate: Thoracic catheters, 5–8 ml hr^{-1}; lumbar catheters, 10–20 ml hr^{-1}.

efferent blockade of sensory, motor and sympathetic nerves, resulting in loss of both sensation and motor control and causes vasodilatation. Dilute local anesthetic solutions given epidurally, provide pain relief and sympathetic blockade without significant motor block. Extremely dilute solutions produce selective analgesia without motor or sympathetic blockade.

The primary reason for using epidural local anesthetics outside the operating room is for the ability to provide the pain relief. Under some circumstances, the sympathetic blockade associated with these agents may also be of benefit in improving tissue perfusion. Further blockade is unneeded and should be avoided.

Once the total mg/hr or μg/hr has been determined, the appropriate volume must be determined to ensure adequate diffusion. Patient age, height and the surgical site all influence the infusion rate; a patient who is 5 feet tall with a lower abdominal incision would require a lower rate than would a patient taller than 6 feet with a thoracotomy incision.

The following concentrations of local anesthetics may be selected:

$$
\begin{aligned}
1/4\% &= 0.25\% &&= 2.5 \text{ mg/ml} \\
1/8\% &= 0.125\% &&= 1.25 \text{ mg/ml} \\
1/10\% &= 0.1\% &&= 1 \text{ mg/ml} \\
1/16\% &= 0.0625\% &&= 0.625 \text{ mg/ml} \\
1/20\% &= 0.05\% &&= 0.5 \text{ mg/ml} \\
1/50\% &= 0.02\% &&= 0.2 \text{ mg/ml} \\
1/100\% &= 0.01\% &&= 0.1 \text{ mg/ml}
\end{aligned}
$$

Patients with a dense sensory or any degree of motor blockade cannot safely ambulate and thus a change to a more dilute (1/20% or less) solution should be made if the patient is ambulatory. Selective blockade achieved with dilute local anesthetics synergize epidural opioid analgesia and provide excellent, selective analgesia. This occurs because pain is modulated differently by these two agents: (a) The opioids modulate via spinal opioid receptors and affect WDR neurons; and (b) the local anesthetic by depolarization of afferent and dorsal horn nociceptive axons and dendrites. Bupivacaine is the primary local anesthetic most often used in combination with epidural opioids because it is most effective in selective blocking of C-fibers in very dilute concentrations. Lidocaine has been used in patients with whom bupivacaine is ineffective, although tachyphylaxis can occur. Chloroprocaine should not be used; it has been suggested that this antagonizes the opioid effect (26).

Always monitor the total dose of narcotic and local anesthetic. Do not exceed 100 μg/hr of fentanyl; 15 mg/hr of meperidine; 1 mg/hr of morphine; or sufentanil 0.3 μg/kg/hr.

PROBLEMS OCCURRING WITH SPINAL OPIOID THERAPY

Side Effects

Respiratory Depression

The incidence of respiratory depression following spinal morphine is 1/10,000 for severe (RR $\leq$ 8) and 1/1000 for mild (RR $\leq$ 12 BPM). Respiratory depression associated with epidural morphine can occur at two different times. "Early" respiratory depression occurs shortly after administration and reflects absorption and circulatory redistribution of the morphine to the brain. It is similar in magnitude to that caused by the same dose administered parenterally. A later, more insidious, "delayed onset" respiratory depression is the result of transport of morphine to brainstem respiratory centers throughout the CSF. In a multicentered study (11) of 14,000 patients treated with epidural morphine, the incidence of significant respiratory depression ranged from 0.25% to 0.40%, with all episodes occurring within 12 hr of administration. Risk factors for the development of significant delayed respiratory depression are outlined in Table 9.3.

Intrathecal administration of morphine was originally associated with higher risk of respiratory depression than with epidural administration. However, with a dose of 1 mg or less the incidence of respiratory depression is similar to that noted with epidural administration.

Although delayed respiratory depression is gradual in onset and reversible with small doses of naloxone, the risk related to this mandates frequent assessment of respiratory status, the use of oxygen saturation monitoring in high risk patients and close observation by the nursing staff. Respiratory rate often does not indicate ventilatory depression; increasing somnolence

TABLE 9.3. *Risk factors for the development of delayed respiratory depression following spinal opioid administration*

Patient related
  Age, >60 years
  Debilitating disease
  Respiratory disease

Drug related
  Hydrophilic opioid (e.g., morphine)
  Large dose of opioid
  Large diluent volume
  Concomitant parenteral opioid administration

Technique related
  Thoracic epidural catheter
  Intrathecal administration
  Position, head of bed <30°

may be a more reliable sign of respiratory compromise and thus the patient's level of consciousness should be closely monitored. Some authors advocate the administration of low dose naloxone or nalbuphine infusions or intermittent doses of naltrexone, as prophylaxis for respiratory depression. However, the incidence of severe respiratory depression is so small that the efficacy of such therapy will likely remain unproven (27).

Rostral spread of lipophilic opioids is less than that of morphine and usually of little clinical significance. Ventilatory compromise is rare and may be related to the concomitant administration of other medications. Early-onset respiratory depression occurs with potent lipophilic opioids, and is the result of vascular uptake and rapid circulation to the brainstem respiratory center. While occasionally severe, such depression is less significant than delayed respiratory compromise, as it is more likely to occur in settings where the patient is closely monitored (operating room, recovery room, Intensive Care Unit), and the anesthesiologist present or readily available to manage the problem.

Nausea and Vomiting

The high incidence of nausea and vomiting noted with intrathecal and epidural administration of opioids is related to rostral CSF transport of opioid molecules to the brainstem's chemoreceptor trigger zone. Nausea is commonly seen in obstetrics, occurring in 20–30% of postcesarean patients treated with epidural morphine. It occurs in approximately 15% of other postoperative patients. Nausea is rarely reported, however, in patients treated with the more lipophilic opioids. In the presence of severe nausea and vomiting, a small bolus of naloxone (40 μg) followed by a continuous infusion 0.5–1 (μg/kg/hr) will attenuate this problem without a significant loss of analgesia. Transdermal scopolamine has also proven effective in this setting but requires 4–6 hr before the maximum benefit is realized (28). Metoclopramide and droperidol are also useful as antiemetics in this setting.

Pruritus

Pruritus is the side effect most commonly seen in patients receiving epidural opioids. Among obstetrical patients, mild pruritus occurs in 70–90% of patients; 45% of surgical patients experience pruritus usually in the face and chest. The cause of pruritus in this setting is not entirely understood, but does not appear to be related to opioid induced histamine release. It may reflect alterations in spinal and trigeminal processing of afferent information, whereby spinal modulation of nociceptive input is reinterpreted as itch at higher centers. Release of histamine at peripheral sites has been suggested to be indirectly linked to changes in spinal efferent outflow.

This would explain why antihistamines provide effective therapy. Other treatments include cold compresses, naloxone infusion (5 μg/kg/hr), and single doses of naltrexone or other opioid agonists/antagonists.

Urinary Retention

Urinary retention most often occurs in young males and has been associated with relaxation of the bladder detrusor muscle. It is rarely seen in obstetrical patients or those receiving long-term epidural opioid therapy. Urinary retention is disturbing to both the patient and surgeon, especially if severe enough to require frequent catheterization or an indwelling catheter. Although the mechanisms underlying urinary retention are not clear, effective therapies include intravenous naloxone and Urecholine.

Breakthrough Pain

The exact nature of "pain" (patient complaint) must first be evaluated. It may not be pain at all, but rather anxiety or other complaints. However, despite the effectiveness of epidural opioids, their use cannot guarantee complete (100%) pain relief.

1. Prior to making any changes in therapy consider:
    a. Increasing the dose of opioid also increases the likelihood of developing sedation, itching, nausea, vomiting, constipation, urinary retention, and respiratory depression.
    b. Increasing the concentration or volume of the local anesthetic delivered may cause areas of numbness with the potential for developing decubiti, as well as be more likely to cause sympathectomy and resultant hypotension.
2. What can be done for breakthrough pain? If analgesia is inadequate, the following should be done:
    a. Verify the functioning of the infusion pump.
    b. Aspirate catheter and check for blood return.
    c. After the application of appropriate monitors, the physician or his/her designate:
        i. Inject 5 ml of 2% lidocaine with epinephrine 1:200,000 (if catheter is thoracic, inject only 3 ml of this solution) to verify catheter location.
        ii. Then, inject 5 to 20 ml of the continuous epidural solution, (dose depends on drug, concentration of solution and placement of catheter) or, 25–100 μg of fentanyl diluted in preservative-free saline may be given (10–20 ml total volume).
    d. If a unilateral block develops, the catheter should be withdrawn 1–2 cm and a second test dose injected.

e. The sudden onset of tachycardia, or the absence of blockade 10–15 min after the catheter is tested, suggests that the catheter has migrated and should be discontinued. A new catheter may be placed after discussion with the Surgical Service.

Anxiety

The use of adjuvant medications in patients receiving spinal opioid analgesia may increase the incidence and severity of respiratory depression and reduce the inherent safety of the therapy. Occasionally, however, sedatives are needed to reduce anxiety or agitation. Benzodiazepines are the most common choice but may themselves cause agitation and confusion, especially in the elderly. Haloperidol is an excellent choice of sedative for elderly patients as it causes less confusion than benzodiazepines. Other useful anxiolytics/sedatives include diphenhydramine, and secobarbital.

Catheter Occlusion

Some causes are epidural catheter kinks, infusion pump inadequacy, presence of particulate substances on the catheter tip, catheter migration, and occlusion at various connector sites.

Epidural catheter kinks should be re-taped. With malfunction of the infusion pump, the pump should be replaced. With occlusion at the connector site, connections should be checked carefully. Occlusive material on the catheter requires flushing the catheter with sterile saline; if the catheter cannot be flushed, it should be discontinued.

Hypotension

Usually hypotension is *not* caused by the infusion mixture. It is a result of *hypovolemia*. It is frequently seen in patients following major abdominal surgery (who have had significant insensible fluid losses. If necessary, stop or decrease the infusion and restart or increase the rate when the fluid deficit is corrected. If there is local anesthetic in the solution, one might also discontinue this.

Other

Disappearing Level

Progressive decline in the level of sensory blockade and ablation of analgesia may be due to a number of phenomena: (a) the infusion pump is off; (b) the tubing is disconnected; (c) the reservoir syringe is empty; or (d) the catheter is no longer in the epidural space.

One must therefore re-check the pump set-up. If this is correct and the pump is functioning properly, then test the catheter to determine its position and location. If the block cannot be reestablished, the catheter should be discontinued. Another catheter may be inserted or alternative analgesia may be initiated.

Dense Motor Blockade

Patients receiving a continuous infusion of 0.25% bupivacaine usually exhibit mild to moderate motor block in the lower extremities. However, if the motor blockade becomes increasingly dense in any patient, suspect subarachnoid migration of the catheter. The catheter should be disconnected from the infusion pump and carefully tested to determine the location.

"Patchy" or Incomplete Block

Attempt to improve the quality of the block by first testing the catheter. If it is properly positioned, administer additional analgesic. The pump should then be reconnected and the infusion rate adjusted upwards as needed.

SUMMARY

Spinal opioid analgesia is an excellent technique for effective and safe relief of postoperative pain. Spinal analgesia decreases morbidity, and the duration of Intensive Care Unit hospital and stays in some patient populations. Certain patient populations (e.g., the elderly or debilitated, patients with extensive systemic disease or those who have undergone extensive or lengthy procedure) may be at an increased risk for respiratory depression. To ensure the safety of these patients, standards for orders, monitoring, and nursing education are imperative. By standardizing care, a consistent and familiar approach to patient management is maintained, and errors of omission or duplication are minimized.

REFERENCES

1. Wang JK, Nauss LA, Thomas JE. Pain relief by intrathecally applied morphine in man. *Anesthesiology* 1979;50:149–150.
2. Cousins MJ, Mather LE. Intrathecal and epidural administration of opioids. *Anesthesiology* 1984;61:276–310.

3. Bromage PR, Camporesi E, Chestnut D. Epidural narcotics for postoperative analgesia. *Anesth Analg* 1980;59:473–480.
4. Yaeger MP, Glass OG, Neff RK. Epidural anesthesia and analgesia in high-risk surgical patients. *Anesthesiology* 1987;66:729–736.
5. Isaacson IJ, Weity FI, Berry AJ, et al. Intrathecal morphine's effect on the postoperative course of patients undergoing abdominal aortic surgery. *Anesth Analg* 1987;66:S86.
6. Duggan AW, Headley PM. Suppression of transmission of nociceptive impulses by morphine. *Br J Pharm* 1977;61:75–76.
7. LaMotte C, Pert CB, Snyder SH. Opiate receptor binding in primate spinal cord: distribution and changes after dorsal roof section. *Brain Research* 1976;112:407–412.
8. Yaksh TL, Rudy TA. Analgesia medicated by a direct spinal action of narcotics. *Science* 1976;192:1357–1358.
9. Yaksh TL. Analgesic actions of intrathecal opiates in cat and primates. *Brain Res* 1978; 153:205–210.
10. Kafen ER, Brown J, Scott D, et al. Bi phasic depression of ventilatory responses to CO_2 following epidural morphine. *Anesthesiology* 1983;58:418–427.
11. Rawal N, Arner S, Gustafsson LL, et al. Present state of extradural and intrathecal opioid analgesia in Sweden. *Br J Anaesthiol* 1987;59:791–799.
12. Birnbach DJ, Arcurio T, Johnson MD, et al. Effect of diluent volume on analgesia produced by epidural fentanyl. *Reg Anesth* 1988;60:13–14.
13. Ready LB, Chadwick HS, Ross B. Age predicts effective epidural morphine dose after abdominal hysterectomy. *Anesth Analg* 1987;66:1215–1218.
14. Gwirtz KH. Intraspinal narcotics in the management of postoperative pain. The Acute Pain Service at Indiana University Hospital. *Anesthesiol Rev* 1990;17:16–28.
15. Yamaguchi H, Watanabe S, Motokawa K, et al. Intrathecal morphine dose response data for pain relief after cholecystectomy. *Anesth Analg* 1990;70:168–171.
16. Wissler RN, Bjoraker DG. Continuous spinal anesthesia microcatheters. *Anesthesiol Rev* 1990;16:49–54.
17. Hunt CO, Naulty JS, Bader AM, et al. Perioperative analgesia with subarachnoid fentanyl-bupivacaine for cesarean delivery. *Anesthesiology* 1989;72:S35–S40.
18. Van den Hooger RH, Colpaert FC. Epidural and subcutaneous morphine, meperidine, fentanyl and sufentanil in the rat. *Anesthesiology* 1987;66:186–194.
20. Glynn CJ, Mather LE, Cousins MJ. Peridural meperidine in humans. *Anesthesiology* 1981;55:520–526.
22. Naulty JS, Barnes D, Becker R, Pate A. Continuous subarachnoid sufentanil for labor analgesia. *Anesthesiology* 1990;73:A964.
23. Naulty JS, Weintraub S, MacMahon J. Epidural butorphanol for post-cesarean delivery pain management. *Anesthesiology* 1984;1:415.
24. Jacobson L, Chabal C, Brody MC, Ward RJ, Ireton RC. Intrathecal methadone and morphine for postoperative analgesia: a comparison of the efficacy, duration, and side effects. *Anesthesiology* 1989;70:742–746.
25. Rosen MA, Dailey PA, Hughes SC, et al. Epidural sufentanil for postoperative analgesia after cesarean section. *Anesthesiology* 1988;68:448–454.
26. Malinow AM, Mokriski BLK, Wakefield ML, et al. Choice of local anesthetic affects post-cesarean epidural fentanyl analgesia. *Reg Anesthiol* 1988;13:141–145.
27. Rawal N, Schott U, Dahlstrom B, et al. Influence of naloxone infusion on analgesia and respiratory depression following epidural morphine. *Anesthesiology* 1986;64:194–201.
28. Loper, KA, Ready LB, Dorman BH. Prophylactic transdermal scopolamine patches reduce nausea in postoperative patients receiving epidural morphine. *Anesth Analg* 1989;68: 144–146.

10

Other Modalities for Acute
Pain Management

The development of Acute Pain Services (APS), with dedicated personnel available to closely observe the patient, allows the use of modalities for postoperative pain management, which have been traditionally used for intraoperative care.

PERIPHERAL NEURAL BLOCKADE

Neural blockade is receiving increasing attention for use in postoperative pain management (1,2). When properly employed, it is a useful tool for managing patients with acute pain. Table 10.1 outlines the basic principles of application, and Table 10.2 reviews continuous regional techniques currently available. Brachial plexus blockade provides upper extremity analgesia via axillary, supraclavicular, or intrascalene approaches. Femoral nerve analgesia may be utilized following surgery on the anterior aspect of the thigh (e.g., skin grafting or saphenous vein stripping) or following lower extremity surgery (e.g., arthroscopy, amputations, knee or ankle surgery). Wound infiltration with 0.5–0.75% bupivacaine with epinephrine 1:200,000 also provide effective analgesia for several hours postoperatively.

The basis for the efficacy and utility of regional nerve blockade in patients with acute pain is by interruption of nociceptive input at its source or by blocking nociceptive transmissions in the peripheral nerve. A thorough knowledge of the pharmacology of local anesthetics is necessary.

Major Nerve Blockade

Brachial Plexus Analgesia

Brachial plexus analgesia in the postoperative setting serve two purposes: (a) pain relief and (b) sympathectomy, which increases extremity blood flow

TABLE 10.1. *Basic principles of application of neural blockade*

Physicians using this method must have ample knowledge of pain syndromes and of all diagnostic and therapeutic measures that can be applied to each patient. Knowledge of advantages, disadvantages, limitations, and complications of each modality provides the broad perspective essential to decide the best therapy or combination of therapies.

Physicians must be willing and able to devote necessary time and effort to evaluate patient through history, general physical, and neurological examination and other studies, event when patient referred by respected colleagues.

Physicians must be highly skilled in the technique and have thorough knowledge of:
Anatomical basis of the procedure
Pharmacology of the local anesthetics
Side effects and possible complications of each procedure and how to prevent and treat
them promptly

Patients must be fully informed of what, how, and why the block is being done:
Unless patients realize the procedure is done only to gain information rather than to cure,
he/she may be disappointed prematurely and refuse to return for further care.
Patients must be assured that all will be done to minimize discomfort.

Careful assessment of patients and results by physician, nurses, and others:
Reaction of the patient to needle insertion and other manipulation to help evaluate "pain
threshold"
Ascertain if intended nerves have been blocked
Evaluate efficacy of block in relieving pain and pathophysiology, and duration for the relief
Record results in detail in patient's chart

Reprinted with permission from reference 1.

TABLE 10.2. *Currently available continuous regional anesthetic techniques by body region*

Body region	Continuous regional anesthetic technique
Head/neck	Cervical plexus block, occipital/nerve block
Upper extremity	Brachial plexus (interscalene block)
Chest wall/upper abdomen	Thoracic epidural catheter, intercostal nerve blocking, interpleural catheter
Lower abdomen/pelvis/ perineum	Lumbar epidural catheter
Lower extremity	Lumbar epidural catheter, lumbar plexus catheter, sciatic perineural catheter, femoral nerve blockade

Reprinted with permission from reference 36.

and may improve surgical outcome in some cases (i.e., digit reimplantation). Analgesia can be obtained using a single dose of local anesthetic injected through a block needle by administering repeated bolus injections or using a continuous infusion of local anesthetic through a catheter placed within the nerve sheath. The choice of local anesthetic for brachial plexus block depends on the duration of blockade needed; lidocaine or mepivacaine provide rapid onset and intermediate duration; bupivacaine and etidocaine provide a longer duration of analgesia.

The brachial plexus can be blocked at a number of different levels (Fig. 10.1). The axillary approach is the most popular. The disadvantage of this approach is that it is inadequate for shoulder procedures. It is, however, the technically easiest of the approaches. The interscalene approach is the recommended site of continuous brachial plexus blockade, as catheters can be secured with less risk of dislodgement or migration than at other sites.

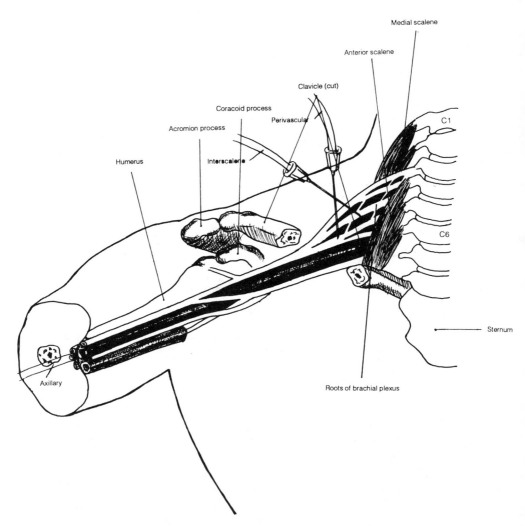

FIG. 10.1. Axillary supraclavicular and intrascalene approaches to brachial plexus analgesia.

Lower Extremity Analgesia

This is usually achieved using major conduction blockade (epidural or spinal). However, as there are only five major nerves supplying the lower extremity, limited analgesia can be achieved by blocking each nerve individually. A sciatic nerve block is useful for postoperative analgesia following procedures on the posterior thigh, lower leg or foot. A femoral nerve block will provide analgesia following saphenous vein stripping, knee arthroscopy or other procedures involving the knee. Both blocks are relatively easy to perform and may significantly decrease parenteral analgesic requirements postoperatively. Selective nerve blockade as opposed to major conduction blockade avoids such problems as urinary retention and hemodynamic changes, associated with spinal analgesia.

Intercostal Nerve Blockade

This block is usually performed at the angle of the rib, lateral to the sacrospinalis muscles and in line with the inferior angle of the scapula (Fig. 10.2). It is a technically easy block, with a success rate approaching 95%. Vascular uptake is extensive and thus epinephrine should be added to solutions of local anesthetic to minimize absorption. This block is extremely effective in providing pain relief for rib fractures, chest tubes and surgical procedures of the upper abdomen and chest.

Infiltrative Techniques

Infiltration, preferably with a long acting local anesthetic such as bupivacaine (0.5–0.75%), is a valuable adjunct for both minor and major surgical procedures. For hernia repairs and excision of minor skin lesions no other analgesia may be necessary. Following arthroscopy or excision of small bony lesions, infiltration may significantly decrease parenteral analgesic use.

Side Effects and Complications of Peripheral Neural Blockade

It deserves emphasis that none of these procedures should be done by staff unable to diagnose and treat complications resulting from the procedure. Moreover, other than infiltration of superficial structures with 3–5 ml of a dilute local anesthetic solution, no block should be performed without intravenous access and the availability of resuscitation equipment.

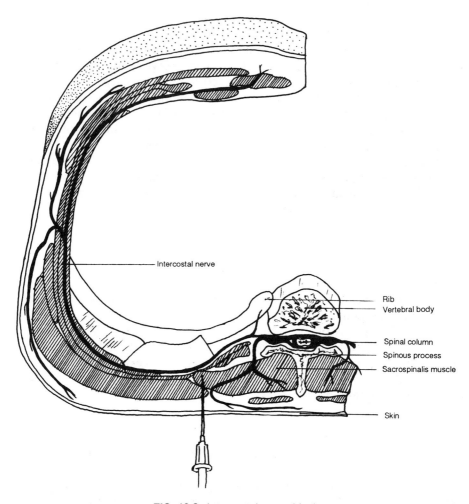

FIG. 10.2. Intercostal nerve block.

Systemic Toxic Reactions

Systemic reactions to local anesthetic result from (a) injection of an excessive dose; (b) inadvertent intravenous injection of a therapeutic dose; and/or (c) abnormal rates of absorption and biotransformation.

Toxic reactions may be arbitrarily classified as mild, moderate and severe. Mild reactions occur when the blood level of the drug is just above physiological limits and may be manifested by palpitations, dryness of the mouth, tinnitus, vertigo, dysarthria, and confusion. Moderate reactions are manifested by severe confusion and muscular twitchings that may progress to convulsions. Severe reactions result from massive overdosage of the drug and are manifested by profound hypotension, bradycardia and respiratory depression which may progress to cardiovascular standstill and respiratory arrest.

Preventive measures include (a) use of the lowest concentration and volume of local anesthetic that assures good analgesia; (b) use of epinephrine containing solutions to retard the rate of local anaesthetic absorption; (c) repeated aspiration prior to each injection to ascertain that the needle tip or catheter is not in a blood vessel; (d) injecting 3 ml of solution as a test dose; if injection is intravascular, the 15 μg of epinephrine in the solution will cause transient tachycardia and hypertension. and (e) injecting large doses of local anesthetic solution in small increments of 3–5 ml to avoid massive intravascular injection.

Treatment of mild reactions includes reassurance to the patient and administration of oxygen. Convulsions must be treated immediately so that the patient does not suffer hypoxia; administer oxygen promptly under positive pressure and control of muscular hyperactivity is by intravenous injection of 40–80 mg of succinylcholine. If any difficulty is encountered in maintaining a patent airway, endotracheal intubation is promptly carried out. Diazepam or thiopental should be given intravenously to control seizure activity. Severe reactions require support of the circulation with fluids and vasopressors, artificial ventilation and CPR if necessary.

High or Total Spinal Anesthesia

High or total spinal anaesthesia and consequent respiratory paralysis and hypotension may develop from inadvertent subarachnoid injections during attempts at interscalene and other nerve blocks in the cervical region. Within a few minutes of injection, there is a rapid development of weakness/sensory loss bilaterally. The patient is restless, drowsy, dyspneic, unable to speak, soon becomes hypoxic and may lose consciousness. Preventive measures include needle insertion perpendicular to the skin in all quadrants; aspiration prior to injection and observing the needle for cerebrospinal fluid backflow after the syringe is detached from the needle.

Treatment consists of (a) endotracheal intubation and ventilation; and (b) support of blood pressure with fluids and intravenous epinephrine as needed.

Pneumothorax

Pneumothorax may occur as a complication of an intercostal nerve block, or infraclavicular, supraclavicular or interscalene brachial plexus block. In experienced hands, the incidence of pneumothorax is usually <1%. Signs and symptoms are usually apparent within a short time of lung puncture but they may not appear until as late as 12 hr after the puncture. A patient with <15–20% pneumothorax may have only mild chest pain, which is accentuated by deep breathing and an occasional cough. With a larger pneumothorax, the pain is more severe and the patient may become dyspneic and hypoxic. A chest X-ray should be taken to confirm the diagnosis and if negative it should be repeated in several hours. Treatment of a small pneumothorax consists of supplemental oxygen, sedation, reassurance, and bedrest. Large pneumothoraces require systemic analgesics, chest tube placement, and the administration of supplemental of oxygen.

Neurological Complications

Gentle contact with a nerve or plexus by the tip of a short bevel block needle may elicit paraesthesia but is very unlikely to result in neurological sequelae. If this does occur after a nerve block, other causes should be considered (3–5). The incidence of persistent nerve injury/dysfunction has been reported to be ≤0.35% (4–8).

If there are repeated insertions of sharp beveled (Quincke tip) needles, or if a intraneural injection occurs, transient nerve dysfunction may develop. In such cases signs of neuropathy may appear between 1 day and up to 1 week after the block, become maximal in about 3 weeks, diminish after 2–3 months. Complete recovery of nerve function usually occurs (9). To minimize the occurrence of this complication it is recommended that short-beveled (45°) needles should be used, that location of the nerve be identified by very gentle paraesthesia or by use of a nerve stimulator and the concentration of the local anaesthetic listed in table should not be exceeded.

INTERPLEURAL ANALGESIA

Interpleural analgesia[1] was described by Reiestad and Stromskag in 1986 (10–12). Since that time the technique has been modified, and it has been shown efficacious for acute pain management.

Overview

Interpleural analgesia is particularly indicated for patients who are at a greater than usual risk for postoperative respiratory insufficiency, due either to pre-existing pathology (e.g., COPD, CHF) or to the surgical procedure

---

[1]The terms interpleural and intrapleural are used interchangeably in the literature. As the catheter placement is between the visceral and parietal pleurae, we have elected to use the terminology interpleural.

itself. Table 10.3 outlines the indications for the use of interpleural analgesia for postoperative pain management.

Patients receiving intrapleural analgesia may have superior postoperative cardiovascular stability (13). This was initially attributed to superior analgesia. However, recent studies suggest the cause is direct blockade of the sympathetic chain and splanchnic outflow leading to sympathetic denervation (13–15). While this technique blunts both visceral and abdominal wall pain, best results might not be achieved without supplemental opioid or anxiolytics. Further study of the effects of interpleural analgesia on the endocrine and stress response is necessary.

Laurito et al. (16) compared the efficacy and safety of continuous infusion versus intermittent bolus injections for postoperative analgesia following cholecystectomy. They reported a more uniform level of pain relief and a reduction in intravenous morphine PCA requirements in the continuous infusion group. Continuous interpleural analgesia has also been shown effective for analgesia in pediatric patients recovering from thoracotomy.

Interpleural analgesia may also provide effective therapy for nonsurgical patients suffering from upper abdominal visceral pain. Durrani et al. (17) recently reported long-lasting pain relief using interpleural injection of 8 ml of 0.5% bupivacaine in patients with upper abdominal pain secondary to pancreatic cancer. This technique may also be useful in patients suffering from pancreatitis (17,18). Contraindications to this technique are outlined in Table 10.4 (18).

General Guidelines

1. Healthcare providers should be familiar with interpleural analgesia: (a) know signs and symptoms of local anesthetic toxicity; (b) know signs and symptoms of pneumothorax; and (c) be knowledgeable about the local anesthetics utilized.

2. Maintain IV access while the interpleural catheter is in place.

3. Obtain a chest X-ray within 1 hr of catheter insertion, and if indicated, within 24 hr of catheter removal.

TABLE 10.3. *Indications for interpleural analgesia in postoperative pain management*

Cholecystectomy
Unilateral breast surgery
Renal surgery
Other subcostal incisions
Thoracotomy
Multiple rib fractures and/or flail chest

Reprinted with permission from Arrow International Inc.

TABLE 10.4. *Contraindications to interpleural analgesia*

PEEP
Pleural fibrosis, pleural adhesions, pleuritis
Pleural effusion
Infection at the insertion site
Allergy to intended local anesthetic
Bullous emphysema
Bleeding diathesis
Recent pulmonary infection

Reprinted with permission from Arrow International Inc.

4. Correct positioning of patient after insertion is critical in determining the extent of the block and pain relief.

5. Problems with injecting through the interpleural catheter include: (a) kinked catheter, either internally or externally; (b) a catheter that is dislodged from the interpleural space; and (c) a filter that is clogged.

Clinical Application

Mode of Action

There are thought to be three different sites of action (19,20): (a) diffusion of local anesthetic from the interpleural space through the parietal pleura and the innermost intercostal muscles to block multiple ipsilateral intercostal nerves; (b) diffusion of the local anesthetic from the pleural space through the most medial portion of the parietal pleural to block the cervical and thoracic portions of the sympathetic chain and the splanchnic nerves; and (c) diffusion of the local anesthetic to the ipsilateral brachial plexus.

The position of the patient after the injection of the local anesthetic determines, to a large part, the nature and extent of the resulting blockade. Many clinicians view the pleural space as a reservoir. By positioning the patient correctly after the injection, the desired blockade will be achieved easily and reliably (10,18) (Figs. 10.3–10.5).

Techniques for Placement

The technique involves the percutaneous placement of a flexible catheter via a thin walled Tuohy needle. A negative pressure gradient (-10 to -12 cm H_2O) is the key to the identification of the pleural space (Figs. 10.6 and 10.7).

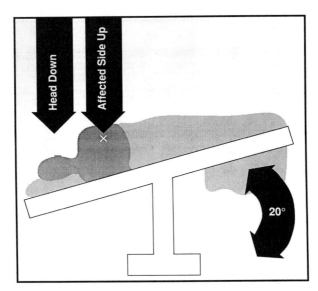

FIG. 10.3. For blockade of the cervical and superior thoracic sympathetic chain, the patient is placed in the lateral decubitus position with the affected side up and trendelenburg for approximately 20–30 min. Reprinted with permission from Arrow International Inc.

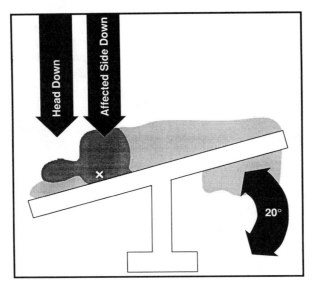

FIG. 10.4. For unilateral block of the intercostal nerves, the patient is placed in the lateral decubitus position with the affected side down and trendelenburg for approximately 20–30 min. Reprinted with permission from Arrow International Inc.

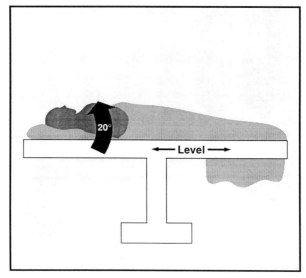

FIG. 10.5. For blockade for postoperative pain management, the patient is placed in a supine position with the bed level. Reprinted with permission from Arrow International Inc.

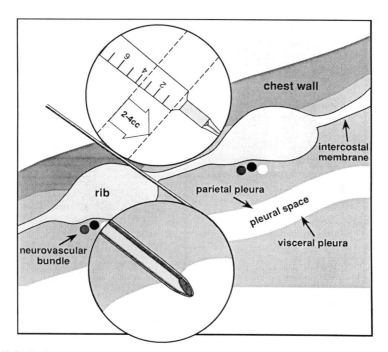

FIG. 10.6. Perforation of the parietal pleura is noted when the negative pressure within the pleural space causes the syringe plunger to advance. Reprinted with permission from Arrow International Inc.

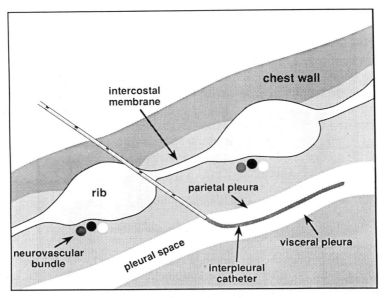

FIG. 10.7. Advance the catheter 5 cm into the pleural space; remove the needle while maintaining catheter position. Reprinted with permission from Arrow International Inc.

Hanging Drop Technique

Recently, Squier et al. (21) described a hanging-drop technique for the identification of the pleural space. After the Tuohy needle is passed superior to the rib, the stylet is removed and the needle is filled with sterile saline until a meniscus is seen at the needle's hub. The needle is then advanced over the edge of the rib until the meniscus disappears when the needle tip enters the interpleural space and the saline is sucked into the space. The catheter is then inserted through the needle and local anesthetic injected through the catheter.

Placement in The Open Chest

Before the thoracotomy incision is closed, the surgeon inserts a Tuohy needle through the skin superior to the rib immediately inferior to the incision while retracting the lung (22–24). The catheter is then passed through the needle and the tip of the catheter is positioned under direct visualization in the paravertebral gutter close to the costovertebral junction. The tip of the catheter is anchored with an absorbable suture so that it remains where positioned in the chest cavity.

Percutaneous Insertion in Children

McIlvaine et al. (25–27) have described an approach to the identification of the pleural space, which is used in spontaneously breathing, anesthetized children. Prior to the termination of the anesthetic, the patient is placed in the lateral decubitus position with the side to be blocked uppermost. An 18-gauge Tuohy needle with a glass syringe attached is inserted through the skin superior to the fourth rib in the midaxillary line. The needle tip is directed in a postero-medial direction to enter the pleural space. The pleural space is identified by the loss of resistance to air, the syringe is then removed and the catheter is threaded 10 cm into the interpleural space. This technique is safe and reliable.

Drugs and Infusion Rates

Interpleural analgesia has greatest benefit when the local anesthetic is administered by an infusion rather than by intermittent boluses given in response to the patient's complaint of pain (28–33).

An initial bolus injection of local anesthetic (usually 30 cc of 0.25% or 0.5% bupivacaine with 1:200,000 epinephrine) is followed by either (a) repeated bolus injections of bupivacaine, with or without epinephrine, 20–30 cc of 0.5% when the patient complains of pain; or, preferably, (b) an infusion of bupivacaine 0.25% with or without epinephrine 1:200,000 at a rate of 10 cc/hr.

With intermittent bolus administration of bupivacaine, the duration of analgesia usually ranges between 6 and 8 hr. Following injection, the patient should be correctly positioned to achieve the desired effect; either supine or with the "affected side down" for 20–30 min (10,18) (Figs. 10.3–10.5).

A continuous infusion provides constant analgesia. Breakthrough pain, however, may occur. It is best alleviated by a change in the patient's position. If repositioning the patient is not effective, supplemental parenteral analgesia may be necessary.

Catheter Care

Infection is very rare (18). A transparent occlusive dressing, such as Tegaderm, should be used over the insertion site. This allows for frequent inspection of the site for signs of infection and extravasation of local anesthetic. If redness, swelling, purulent drainage, or fever occurs, the APS physician should be notified immediately. To minimize the risk of infection: (a) A catheter should not be inserted through infected skin. (b) Strict aseptic technique should be maintained. (c) The catheter, tubing, and pump should be labeled properly. (d) The filters and injection caps should be changed at least every 72 hr. (e) If an intermittent bolus technique is utilized, cleanse the injection cap prior to administration; if a continuous infusion is utilized ensure all connections are secure. (f) Assess the catheter insertion site at least once a shift for signs of infection.

Complications

Pneumothorax

This is the most common of the potentially serious complications. The incidence is reportedly between 1% and 5%. One must differentiate a pneumothorax from the small amount of air introduced with insertion which may be seen on chest X-ray over the apex of the lung. This air is not leaking from an injured lung, but is air entrained while the technique is being performed and can usually be aspirated through the interpleural catheter. If this air does not clear with aspiration, it *should not* be treated with the insertion of a chest tube; as this is harmless, the air is rapidly absorbed and it will not expand.

If, however, a puncture of the lung occurs, it may require intervention. A <10% pneumothorax will resolve in 24–48 hr, and requires no intervention. A significant (>10%) pneumothorax, however, may necessitate insertion of a chest tube for 2–3 days (10,12,18).

Infection

Bacterial infection at the insertion site may lead to the development of an empyema or bronchopleural fistula. Infection is very rare and can be avoided by adhering to strict sterile insertion technique.

Trauma to the Neurovascular Bundle

This is an uncommon complication. The catheter is placed superior to the rib margin, away from the intercostal vessels and nerve.

Systemic Local Anesthetic Toxicity

Local anesthetic toxicity is most likely to occur with the injection of a large amount of concentrated local anesthetic. A volume of 20–30 ml of 0.5% bupivacaine with or without epinephrine should not result in toxic blood levels (15). Central nervous system toxicity has occurred in one patient (27) who had a recent history of pneumonia. This may have been secondary to a more rapid systemic absorption of the local anesthetic from the infected area.

Allergic Reactions

Sensitivity to local anesthetics may manifest itself as an allergic dermatitis, a bronchospasm, or an anaphylactic reaction. Lidocaine and bupivacaine, the most commonly used local anesthetics for interpleural analgesia, are amides and rarely cause allergic reactions.

TRANSDERMAL DRUG DELIVERY

At the present time, transdermal drug delivery systems are available for administering scopolamine, estradiol, nitroglycerine, and, of interest in acute pain management, fentanyl and clonidine.

Delivery of drugs through the skin utilizes the properties of the stratum corneum, which slows down the entry of drug into the circulation. The skin not only governs drug release from the external reservoir, but may itself act as a reservoir or depot for secondary drug release. This skin reservoir causes a time delay until the adequate plasma drug concentration is reached. It is important in causing the plateau effect, which allows a constant plasma drug concentration in patients receiving transdermal medication. The penetration rate, or flux, of different substances may vary by orders of magnitude. One can, however, generalize the following: (a) High molecular weight polymers and macromolecules penetrate poorly. (b) Water-soluble electrolytes penetrate poorly. (c) Lipid-soluble substances penetrate best, especially if moderate molecular weight and nonpolar. In addition, physical characteristic of the stratum corneum affect permeability (Table 10.5).

Transdermal Fentanyl

Transdermal fentanyl (TTS Fentanyl-Duragesic) is approved for use in chronic pain. At at present FDA approval for application in acute pain is pending.

The transdermal therapeutic system (TTS) developed by Alza Corporation for fentanyl delivery has a microporous membrane which is designed to be the rate-limiting step in drug transfer. The variability in absorption rate related to the skin factors is reduced (Table 10.5) The TTS fentanyl patch is a rectangular, transparent unit comprising four function layers: (a) a backing layer of polyester film, (b) a drug reservoir of fentanyl and alcohol in a gel matrix which incidentally makes the potential for extraction and abuse minimal, (c) a copolymer membrane that controls fentanyl delivery to the skin surface, and (d) a silicane adhesive (Fig 10.8).

TABLE 10.5. *Factors affecting skin permeability*

Body site
Skin temperature
Ethnic group
Skin damage
Chemicals
Degree of hydration

Reprinted with permission from reference 34.

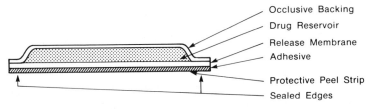

FIG. 10.8. Transdermal delivery system.

TTS fentanyl is available in four different sizes to allow drug release at four different rates: 10, 20, 30, and 40 cm^2 which release drug at 25, 50, 75, or 100 μg/hr. The drug per unit area is identical in all four patch sizes: Each 10 cm^2 contains 2.5 mg fentanyl + (0.1 ml alcohol), and releases fentanyl at 25 μg/hr. Each patch provides its continuous dose for 72 hr.

Studies (34) thus far have shown TTS fentanyl to be efficacious and as safe as other types of opioid analgesia for postoperative pain. However, due to the long time required to reach therapeutic plasma levels, additional analgesics must be available for the first 12–18 hr. TTS fentanyl is thus likely to remain an adjunctive therapy or to be used when PCA therapy is unavailable or contraindicated.

Transdermal Clonidine

Alpha-2 adrenergic agonists (Transdermal clonidine; Catapres TTS) have been used by many investigators to decrease intraoperative anesthetic requirements. Shafer et al. have extended the use of the transdermal preparation into the postoperative period and have shown lower postoperative narcotic requirements. This preparation has signified potential as an alternative and/or adjuvant to opioids for postoperative pain management. Like other transdermal preparation, the time from application to therapeutic plasma levels is long; a single dose of oral clonidine administered at the time of patch application, which is ideally 8–12 hr preoperatively should eliminate this time postoperatively when plasma levels are not adequate.

NONSTEROIDAL ANTIINFLAMMATORY DRUGS

Nonsteroidal antiinflammatory drugs (NSAIDs) are useful in a variety of clinical situations, including the treatment of inflammatory joint disease and myalgias, and as adjuvants for surgical cancer and traumatic pain (35). Their antipyretic and platelet-aggregation inhibiting effects are also useful. NSAIDs are felt to produce analgesia primarily by their ability to prevent elaboration of prostaglandins, thus preventing nociceptor sensitization and lowering the pain threshold. Acting at the periphery, NSAIDs act additively with opioids, which act centrally, to inhibit afferent nociceptor input.

NSAIDs differ from opioid analgesics in that there is a ceiling effect to analgesia; they do not produce tolerance or physical or psychologic dependence. It is difficult to determine which NSAID the individual patient will best respond to or tolerate.

Nonanalgesic effects and side effects to consider when using NSAIDs include the following: (a) NSAIDs inhibit platelet aggregation by reversibly inhibiting prostaglandin synthetase. Therefore, the concomitant use of anticoagulation is a relative contraindication to their use. Aspirin irreversibly inhibits prostoglandin synthetase. (b) They are ulcerogenic; patients with a history of peptic ulcer disease, debilitating diseases, and advanced age appear to be the most susceptible. (c) They can produce renal insufficiency: They decrease synthesis of renal vasodilator prostaglandins, may cause interstitial nephritis, they may impair renin secretions and enhanced tubular water and sodium reabsorption. The following should be noted:
1. Interstitial nephritis is idiosyncratic and generally reversible with discontinuation of the drug.
2. Papillary necrosis is primarily associated with phenacetin.
3. These agents can also affect liver function. While clinically significant effects rarely occur in normal patients, all NSAIDs can elevate liver enzymes. They can also reduce the levels of vitamin K dependent clotting factors. Hepatic toxicity is more likely in the presence of advanced age (related to decreased drug metabolism), decreased renal clearance, prolonged therapy at high dose, and multiple drug use; patients with juvenile rheumatoid arthritis, rheumatic fever, or systemic lupus are at increased risk.

(d) The drug interactions are as follows: cimetidine may increase its half-life; mildly hypertensive subjects showed a mild decrease in the hypotensive effect of a single dose of propranolol but not of atenolol; and NSAID's can increase lithium levels by as much as 22%, with toxicity characterized by symptoms of polyuria, muscular weakness, lethargy and tremors. Serum lithium levels should be monitored closely, with the doses adjusted accordingly.

ORAL OPIOID PREPARATIONS

Methadone

Methadone is primarily a mu agonist with pharmacological properties qualitatively similar to those of morphine. The onset of analgesia occurs 10–20 min following administration. Despite its longer plasma half-life, the duration of the analgesic action of single doses is essentially the same as that of morphine. Oral methadone can be used as maintenance for an opioid tolerant individual using shorter acting preparations for acute pain requirements. It can take the place of a continuous opioid infusion in patients with severe pain (sickle cell crisis, major orthopedic procedures).

MS Contin

MS Contin is useful when parenteral opioid requirements are high postoperatively. Like oral methadone, it can take the place of a continuous opioid infusion.

TRANSCUTANEOUS ELECTRICAL NERVE STIMULATION

Transcutaneous electrical nerve stimulation (TENS) is a safe, noninvasive, drug-free method of pain management. TENS is believed to relieve pain by blocking nociceptic afferent input to the brain and by activation of endorphin release. TENS is most commonly utilized for chronic pain management, but has gained respect in the acute postoperative setting as an adjunct to opioid therapy.

CRYOANALGESIA

Cryoanalgesia is a technique that has had limited utilization in acute postoperative pain management. It has primarily been used for post-thoracotomy pain. The analgesia is often incomplete, often requiring supplemental analgesia. Problems such as unwanted chest wall bleeding; potential damage to surrounding tissues and post-procedural neuralgias have been described (36).

ADJUVANT MEDICATIONS

Anxiolytics

Anxiolytics are effective for treatment of acute anxiety and muscle spasm (diazepam) with postoperative pain. These agents have no analgesic properties. However, because of their sedative and respiratory depressant effects, the amount of opioid given may need to be decreased when these are added.

Antidepressants

Antidepressants are frequently used to treat neuropathic pain that has been caused by surgical trauma, radiation therapy, chemotherapy, or malignant nerve infiltration. Amitriptyline has the best documented analgesia, but it is the least tolerated because of its potent anticholinergic effects. Sedation and orthostatic hypotension are also frequent, and may limit the concomitant use of opioid analgesic. They can also affect the perception of pain or mood.

Antihistamines

Hydroxyzine has analgesic, antiemetic, and mild sedative activity in addition to its antihistamine effects. It augments opioid analgesia, and is a useful adjuvant for the anxious or nauseated patient.

Barbiturates

Barbiturates do not have intrinsic analgesic properties and should be avoided in the management of pain.

Phenothiazines

Phenothiazines can be used to prevent opioid-induced nausea. They may exacerbate the hypotensive and sedating effects of opioids and should be used with care.

Anticonvulsants

Anticonvulsants are useful for pain arising from peripheral nerve syndromes.

SUMMARY

The clinician should be aware of all modalities available for postoperative pain management and be guided by the clinical situation to determine appropriate pain management for the individual patient.

REFERENCES

1. Bonica FF. Local anaesthesia and regional blocks. In: Wall PD, Melzack R, eds. *Textbook of Pain*. 2nd ed. New York: Churchill Livingstone, 1984.
2. Cousins MJ, Brigenbaugh PO, eds. *Neural blockade in clinical anesthesia and management of pain*. 2nd Edition. Philadelphia: J.B. Lippincott, 1988.
3. Dhuner KG. Nerve injures following operations. A survey of cases occurring during a 6 year period. *Anesthesiology* 1950;11:289–293.
4. Bonica JJ. *Management of pain*. 2nd ed. Philadelphia: Lea and Febiger. 1990.
5. Swerdlow M. Complications of local anesthetic neural blockade. In: Cousins MJ, Bridenbaugh PO, eds. *Neural blockade in clinical anesthesia and management of pain*. Philadelphia: JB Lippincott, 1980.
6. Moore DC. Regional block, 4th edition, Springfield, IL: Charles C. Thomas, 1965.
7. Moore DC. Complications of regional anesthesia. In: Bonica JJ, ed. *Regional anesthesia*. Philadelphia: FA Davis, 1971.
8. Winchell SW, Wolfe R. The incidence of neuropathology following upper extremity blocks. *Reg Anaesthiol* 1985;10:12–15.
9. Lofstrom B, Wennberg A, Widen L. Late disturbances in nerve function after block with local anaesthetic agents. *Acta Anaesthiol Scand* 1966;10:111–122.
10. Reiestad, F, Stromksag KE. Intrapleural catheter in management of postoperative pain. *Anesthesiology* 1986;11:89–90.
11. Kvalheim L, Reiestad F. Intrapleural catheter in the management of postoperative pain. *Anesthesiology* 1984;61:A231.
12. Riestad F, Stromskag KE. Interpleural catheter in the management of postoperative pain. A preliminary report. *Reg Anesthiol* 1989;68:5228.
13. Seltzer JL, Larijani GE, Goldberg ME, Marr A. Intrapleural bupivacaine—a kinetic and dynamic evaluation. *Anesthesiology* 1987;67:798–800.
14. Agostini E. Mechanics of the pleural space. *Physiol Rev* 1972;52:57–128.
15. Covino BG. Interpleural regional analgesia [Editorial]. *Anesth Analg* 1988;67:427–429.
16. Laurito CE, Riegler FX, Vadeboncover TR, et al. Does a continuous infusion of intrapleural bupivacaine optimize post cholecystectomy pain? *Anesth Analg* 1990;70:S450.
17. Durrani Z, Winnie AP, Ikuta P. Interpleural catheter analgesia for pancreatic pain. *Anesth Analg* 1988;67:479–481.
18. Reiestad F. Interpleural regional analgesia—a new method for pain relief in various acute and chronic pain conditions [Thesis summary]. Department of Anesthesia, Ulleval University Hospital, Oslo, Norway, 1989.
19. Camporesi E. Intrapleural analgesia: a new technique. *J Cardiothorac Anesthiol* 1989; 3:137–138.
20. Schlesinger TM, Laurito CE, Baughman VL, Carranza CJ. Interpleural bupivacaine for mammography during needle localization and breast biopsy. *Anesth Analg* 1989;68: 394–395.
21. Squier RC, Morrow JS, Roman R. Hanging drop technique for intrapleural analgesia. *Anesthiology* 1989;70:822.
22. Chan VWS, Arthur GR, Ferrante FM. Intrapleural bupivacaine administration for pain relief following thoracotomy. *Regional Anesthiol* 1988;13:2S;70.
23. Chan V, Chung F, Cheng DCH, Kirby TJ, Chung A, Sandler A. Continuous intercostal nerve block for pain relief following thoracotomy—a new approach. *Canadian J Anesthiol* 1988;35:S113–S114.

24. El-Baz N, Faber LP, Ivankovich AD. Intrapleural infusion of local anesthetic: a word of caution [Letter]. *Anesthesiology* 1988;68:809–810.
25. McIlvaine WB, Knox RF, Fennessey PV, Goldstein M. Continuous infusion of bupivacaine via intrapleural catheter for analgesia after thoracotomy in children. *Anesthesiology* 1988;69:261–264.
26. McIlvaine WB, Chang JT, Jones M. The effective use of intrapleural bupivacaine for analgesia after thoracic and subcostal incision sin children. *J Pediatr Surg* 1988;12:1184–1187.
27. Queen JS, Kahana MD, DiFazio CA, et al. An evaluation of interpleural analgesia with etidocaine in children. *Anesth Analg* 1989;68:S228.
28. Brismar B, Pettersson N, Tokis L, Strandberg A, Hedenstierna G. Postoperative analgesia with intrapleural administration of bupivacaine-adrenaline. *Acta Anesthesiol Scand* 1987;31:515–520.
29. Kamban Jr, Jammon J, Parris WCV, Lupinetti FM. Intrapleural analgesia for post-thoracotomy pain and blood levels of bupivacaine following intrapleural injection. *Can J Anesthiol* 1989;36:106–109.
30. Rosenberg PH, Scheinin BM-A, Lepantalo MJA, Lindors O. Continuous intrapleural infusion of bupivacaine for analgesia after thoracotomy. *Anesthesiology* 1987;67:811–813.
31. Jorfeldt L, Lofstrom B, Pernow B, Persson B, Wahren J, Widman B. The effects of local anesthetics on the central circulation and respiration in man and dog. *Acta Anesthesiol Scand* 1968;12:153–169.
32. Ryan DW. Accidental intravenous injection of Bupivacaine: A complication of obstetrical epidural anesthesia. *Br J Anesth* 1973;45:907–908.
33. Stromskag KE, Reiestad F, Holmqvist ELO, Ogenstad S. Intrapleural administration of 0.25%, 0.375% and 0.5% bupivacaine with epinephrine after cholecystectomy. *Anesth Analg* 1988;67:430–443.
34. Shafer SL. Transdermal opioids in postoperative pain. *Anesthesiol Rep* 1990;2:176–186.
35. Fragen RJ. NSAIDs in acute postoperative pain control. *Anesthesiol Rep* 1990;2:187–192.
36. Lee VC. Non-narcotic modalities for the management of acute pain. In: Benumof JL, Oden RV, eds. *Management of postoperative pain. Anesthesiology clinics of North America.* 1989;7:1:63–78.

11

Acute Pain Management for Specific Patient Populations

Linda M. Preble and Raymond S. Sinatra

Physicians routinely alter the doses of opioids, based on the physical condition and characteristics of the patient (1). Age, gender, concomitant medications, and the operative site will all affect opioid requirements. There is no correlation between analgesic requirements and weight, height, or body surface area; these factors do influence serum opioid concentration. However, circulating blood levels are not directly related to analgesic effects (2). Burns et al. (3) studied the influence of patient characteristics on the requirements for postoperative analgesia and found that males required a significantly greater amount of opioids in the first 24 hr following surgery than females. Patient age appears to be the most important variable in determining the degree of pain relief achieved from a dose of opioid (4). Burns et al. (3), however, found that there was no correlation between age and the *level* of pain relief, but a significant decrease in consumption of opioids with increasing age was noted. Furthermore, the dose and volume of injectate utilized to achieve pain relief with epidural/spinal opioid administration is influenced by age. Obviously individualization of analgesic therapy is crucial if the clinician hopes to improve postoperative pain management (5). The only safe and effective way to administer an opioid analgesic is to observe the individual's response (6).

The purpose of this chapter is to provide guidelines for the management of pain in various clinical settings. The mental and physical capabilities of the patient, as well as the factors discussed above, will influence the choice of analgesic therapy.

OBSTETRICS

Pain management for the postoperative obstetrical patient presents a unique challenge. The patient needs adequate pain therapy, while at the same time she wants to be alert and able to interact with her newborn. The effect of medication on the newborn given to the nursing mother must also be considered.

PCA

Patient-controlled analgesia (PCA) is ideally suited for use in postcesarean patients. It provides effective analgesia with minimal sedation. Sinatra et al. (7) demonstrated the effectiveness of PCA in this setting. In a double-blinded randomized study, PCA morphine, oxymorphone, and meperidine were evaluated in this patient population. The results showed that while all three treatment groups reported excellent analgesia, those receiving oxymorphone and meperidine reported lower pain scores at rest, had less sedation, and reported a higher satisfaction than patients treated with morphine. The patients receiving oxymorphone had significantly less pain with movement. Patients treated with meperidine had minimal sedation and the lowest incidence of side effects. There are, however, disadvantages to utilizing meperidine in the obstetrical setting. Its metabolite, norme-peridine, concentrates in breast milk. In a recent evaluation of infants of nursing mothers (8), neonatal neurobehavior (as assessed by the Brazelton Neonatal Behavioral Assessment Scale), in those infants whose mothers were utilizing PCA meperidine for postcesarean analgesia, were lower than those of mothers who were utilizing morphine. The results of this prelimi-nary study suggests that meperidine may not be the drug of choice in nursing mothers. Furthermore, normeperidine is epileptogenic. Thus, its use in the patient with pregnancy induced hypertension is questionable because of the greater risk of seizures in the population.

Of the other PCA opioids available, oxymorphone is associated with a high incidence of nausea and vomiting, which is an unacceptable side effect in this patient population. Morphine produces a significant degree of seda-tion, has a slow onset, and was not shown as effective for pain relief as oxymorphone. Hydromorphone has been shown a better analgesic than meperidine (9), and may be the drug of choice in this patient population.

Spinal Opioids

Epidural opioids provide superior analgesia in this population (10). For continuous epidural infusion, lipophilic agents, such as fentanyl or sufentanil with or without dilute bupivacaine (1/8%, 1/16%) is preferable. They have a rapid onset and a short duration, which makes them ideally suited for continuous epidural infusion techniques, where the level of anal-gesia can be carefully titrated to the level of pain stimulus and the effect can be rapidly terminated if problems should occur.

Morphine is the drug of choice for a single dose injection, providing effective analgesia for 18–24 hr. It is, unfortunately, associated with a high incidence of pruritus (60–90%), nausea, and urinary retention. Furthermore, there is always the risk of significant respiratory depression, although this population is at low risk for this complication (11). Harrison et al. (10) conducted a controlled randomized study comparing IV-PCA morphine and epidural morphine (5 mg). Patients receiving epidural morphine, while benefiting from a significantly improved level of analgesia, were troubled by a high incidence of pruritus (70%), which was often severe enough to require treatment. Despite lower pain scores than obtained by those receiving IV-PCA morphine, patient satisfaction with epidural morphine analgesia was less than with IV-PCA morphine. The lack of troublesome side effects, and the ability to self administer analgesia appears to make IV-PCA the preferred pain therapy in postcesarean patients.

PCA in many institutions may not be instituted immediately postoperative. Therefore, analgesia in that "transitional" period must be addressed. In our institution, spinal meperidine (50 mg epidural or 10 mg intrathecal) is given to provide approximately 4–6 hr of analgesia and allow transition to IV-PCA without side effects or the need for other medication.

GYNECOLOGY

PCA

PCA is ideally suited for use in gynecological patients. It provides effective analgesia with a minimum degree of sedation, allowing for early ambulation and an improved postoperative course (12). Opioids, however, appear to contribute to the high incidence of postoperative nausea and vomiting seen in this population. The application of transdermal scopolamine appears to significantly reduce the incidence of nausea and vomiting in this patient population (13). The addition of promethazine to PCA morphine also appears to reduce the severity of nausea and vomiting without increasing the level of sedation (14).

GUIDELINES FOR THE CHOICE OF OPIOID

Meperidine

Meperidine appears to best treat visceral/spasmodic pain, which may be seen in patients who have had manipulation of the ovaries and tubes. We elect meperidine in this population.

Morphine

Morphine produces excellent analgesia in this population. The sedation seen in the obstetrical setting is not a problem in gynecological patients.

Hydromorphone

Hydromorphone provides excellent analgesia. However, large PCA bolus doses (0.2 mg or higher) increase the incidence of nausea and vomiting.

Oxymorphone

Oxymorphone increases the incidence of nausea and vomiting. A significant drawback to this drug is its high cost.

Spinal Opioids

Epidural opioids provide superior analgesia in this patient population. Institutional policy will govern whether or not a patient is discharged to the postoperative ward with the epidural catheter in place. This will influence the drug of choice utilized for postoperative pain management.

Morphine

Morphine provides effective analgesia for 12–24 hr. However, it is associated with a high incidence of severe pruritus (60–90%), nausea, and urinary retention, which may be treated with naloxone infusions. Furthermore, there is always a risk of respiratory depression, especially in the elderly/debilitated patient. Thus, patients with high risk for respiratory depression should receive spinal morphine only if they will be in a monitored setting (i.e., Intensive Care Unit).

Meperidine

Single doses of meperidine provide 4–6 hr of analgesia and smooth the transition onto PCA. Continuous meperidine (or meperidine-bupivacaine) infusions may also be utilized.

Lipophilic Agents

For epidural infusion, lipophilic agents, such as fentanyl or sufentanil with or without dilute bupivacaine (1/8%, 1/10%, 1/16%), are effective in these patients.

ORTHOPEDICS

Orthopedic patients may suffer from severe pain that is often difficult to treat with parenterally administered opioids. The nature of surgery affects postoperative opioid requirements and will influence the modality chosen (Table 11.1).

PCA

Morphine and hydromorphone are the PCA drugs of choice in orthopedics. The degree of pain relief offered by meperidine is often insufficient.

A basal infusion of opioid (equivalent to 50–100% of the PCA bolus dose/hour) is often employed during the first 24 hr following surgery. NSAIDs, either orally, intramuscularly, or intravenously, provide effective supplementation of PCA opioid therapy and may reduce or eliminate the need for a basal infusion.

Spinal Opioids

Spinal analgesia may be of benefit in patients with very high narcotic requirements (e.g. as following total knee reconstruction). Epidurally administered morphine or fentanyl, combined with dilute concentrations of bupivacaine (1/10% or less), provide excellent analgesia for lower extremity

TABLE 11.1. *Postoperative opioid requirements for orthopedic surgery*

	VAS pain			Narcotic (average dose/hr)	Age in years (mean ± SD)
	Mean ± SD	Mean	Range		
Anterior Cruciate Ligament Repair	5.0 ± 1.4	4	4–7	4.6 ± 1.6	26 ± 7.1
Ankle	6.3 ± 1.9	6	4–10	3.4 ± 1.6	48.4 ± 17.5
Femur	5.9 ± 2.5	5	2–10	3.6 ± 2.8	34.2 ± 16.1
Back Fusion	6.2 ± 2	6	3–9	5.4 ± 4.8	33.6 ± 8.9
Hip	2.6 ± 1.9	3	0–6	1.2 ± 1	67 ± 12.3
Lami	4.4 ± 2.3	5	3–10	2.8 ± 2	49.6 ± 13.7
Tibia	4.8 ± 1.9	5.5	2–6	3.0 ± 0.4	22.8 ± 1.6
Total Knee Replacment	5.3 ± 3	5.5	0–10	2.1 ± 0.8	61.7 ± 16.4

Reproduced with permission from Harris SN, Sevarino FB, Silverman DS, et al. Prophylactic transdermal scopolamine for patients using patient controlled analgesia. Anesthesiology, 1989; 71:3A690.

orthopedic surgery. This technique is unfortunately associated with a high incidence or urinary retention, often requiring catheterization and thus places the patient, especially one with prosthetics, at a greater risk for infection. For this reason, the technique should be reserved for high-risk patients where benefits of a greater intensity of analgesia outweigh the side effects.

Peripheral Nerve Blocks/Local Infiltration

Peripheral nerve blockade is an underused technique in this population. It offers intense analgesia although it is often associated with motor blockade (see Chapter 10). Consider this technique where appropriate.

GENERAL SURGERY

The nature of surgery, as well as the surgical site, will influence the choice of postoperative pain therapy. Patients who have undergone simple urologic procedures, (e.g., transurethral prostatectomy, cystoscopies, or ureteral stone extraction) or simple general surgical procedures, (e.g., simple mastectomies) achieve good pain relief with conventional analgesics. Patients who have undergone extensive surgical procedures (e.g., retropubic prostatectomies, nephrectomies, bowel resections, liver resections) will require more aggressive pain management.

Morbidly obese and other high-risk patients treated with PCA, spinal, or interpleural analgesia should be monitored using pulse oximetry or apnea monitoring, and will often require an Intensive Care Unit as well.

PCA

PCA is most effective in smaller, less traumatic surgical procedures. It is also the choice in cases where anticoagulation or other factors contraindicate spinal analgesia. Morphine and hydromorphone are the preferred opioids for extensive incisional and/or deep muscle-related pain. However, morphine can increase vasovagal reactions, increase the incidence of urinary retention in elderly males, and increase smooth muscle spasm in patients who have had ureteral manipulation or cholecystectomies. Meperidine may be the preferred opioid for controlling the intermittent spasmodic pain seen following ureteral surgery or cholecystectomy.

Spinal Opioids

Spinal opioids (intermittent bolus, single dose, or continuous infusions) are recommended in high-risk patients, as they offer superior analgesia when compared to parenteral opioids. When properly administered, intrathecal and epidural opioids can, in many cases, prevent the pain stimulus from being perceived, minimize deterioration of pulmonary function, and limit sympathoadrenal responses (1,2,15).

Morphine is the preferred opioid for patients recovering from large incisions and massive tissue injury. However, the segmental analgesia provided by the lumbar administration of lipophilic agents is useful in lower abdominal areas. When lipophilic agents are administered via thoracic catheters, analgesia is adequate for upper abdominal or thoracic incisions as well. Monitoring should be determined by the medical condition of the patient; those patients who are at a great risk of respiratory depression (see Chapter 9) should be monitored closely. Low-dose naloxone (40–80 μg/hr) infusions can be used to reduce the risk of respiratory depression and to reduce the incidence of side effects, in particular, pruritus and urinary retention.

Interpleural Analgesia

Interpleural analgesia provides excellent analgesia for patients who have had flank incisions (e.g., nephrectomy, cholecystectomy), unilateral breast surgery, and subcostal incisions. The patients are at more than the usual risk for postoperative respiratory insufficiency secondary to splinting related to the pain of the surgical incision. Contraindications to this technique are discussed in Chapter 10.

CARDIOTHORACIC

The adverse effects of pain can be deleterious after cardiac surgery. Pain stimulates the autonomic nervous systems, which increase sympathetic tone and leads to a release of cathecholamines, with resultant increase in total peripheral vascular resistance, heart rate, myocardial contractility, myocardial oxygen consumption, and possibly produce tachydysrhythmias (16).

PCA

PCA is not appropriate for confused, disoriented, physically incapacitated, or intubated patients. The anesthetic for cardiac surgery commonly involves the use of moderate to high doses of intravenous opioids, which usually result in postoperative ventilation for 12–24 hr. Thus, PCA is inappropriate in the immediate postoperative period.

Most patients undergoing thoracic surgery are extubated at the conclusion of the procedure. Thus, PCA would provide the means for the patient to self administer pain medication and allow greater individualization of therapy. Morphine and hydromorphone are preferred for these patients.

Spinal Analgesia

Analgesia following cardiac and thoracic surgery may be optimally achieved with spinal opioids. The risk of epidural hematoma related to heparization for cardiopulmonary bypass was addressed by Tuman (14), who concluded that epidural or intrathecal analgesia is safe and was not associated with epidural hematomas in over 4,000 patients who were anticoagulated for their surgical procedure. This technique must still be used with great forethought and caution in patients who will undergo cardiopulmonary bypass.

For thoracic surgical procedures, spinal opioids provide the most optimal pain relief especially when the catheter is inserted at the level of the incision. El-Bas (17) studied continuous epidural infusion of morphine for the treatment of pain after thoracic surgery and showed effective pain relief with this technique. Cullen (18) determined that the addition of bupivacaine to morphine epidural infusions provided better relief of pain than morphine alone. Fisher (19) noted the presence of buttock numbness (61%) and leg weakness (74%) in patients receiving continuous epidural infusions with fentanyl (10 mcg/ml) and bupivacaine (0.1%) or morphine (0.1 mg/ml) and bupivacaine (0.1%) at a rate of 5 ml/hr. This incidence may be reduced by diluting the local anesthetic concentration below 0.1%. Lipophilic agents may be utilized for thoracic incisional pain relief. They are most effective when the catheter is inserted at the thoracic level. Inadequate pain relief is not uncommon when attempting to achieve pain relief at a thoracic level with a catheter inserted at a lumbar site.

Interpleural Analgesia

Interpleural analgesia provides excellent analgesia for patients who have had thoracotomy incisions, and can decrease the risk of postoperative respiratory insufficiency and atelectasis. For interpleural analgesia to be most effective, the chest tube must be clamped for approximately 20–30 min after a bolus injection. The efficacy of interpleural analgesia using a continuous infusion technique in the patient with a chest tube has not been well defined.

In summary, pain after cardiothoracic surgery may be minimal or may result in severe physiologic changes that are detrimental to the patient. Each method of analgesia has advantages and disadvantages. The choice of which modality to use depends on the skill of the clinician and institutional practices.

VASCULAR SURGERY

Analgesic requirements initially will depend upon what intraoperative anesthetic technique was used (20). Whatever the intraoperative management, eventually there will be a need for additional analgesics in the postoperative period.

PCA

Spinal opioids provide superior pain relief in vascular surgery and are recommended whenever available. There is no clear opioid preference if this modality is used.

Spinal Opioids

Spinal opioids provide excellent analgesia, minimize the stress response to surgery, reduce the excess antidiuretic hormone production, and reduce the excess urinary excretion of cortisol, catecholamines and nitrogen (20). Unfortunately, the controversy related to heparinization again arises in this patient population. The risk of the development of an epidural hematoma associated with heparinization is of concern with respect to the spinal or epidural analgesia in this population.

Spinal opioids appear to be associated with a lower procedure-related morbidity. Their use is justified, despite the theoretical risk of epidural hematoma (20).

The use of continuous local anesthetic infusion is not optimal in vascular surgery patients because of the disturbance of the autonomic control of blood pressure which epidurally applied local anesthetics produce (21). The optimal choice is the combination of opioid and dilute local anesthetic continuous infusion.

PEDIATRICS

A child's perception of pain closely parallels his/her intellectual and social development. In the past, postsurgical pediatric patients have generally been undermedicated, as they were believed to be highly sensitive to opioid analgesics and/or not experience pain. In recent years, pain management has become a priority in the perioperative management of the pediatric patient.

Non-opioid Analgesics

Nonopioid analgesics are useful for treatment of mild to moderate pain or as an adjuvant to opioid therapy. With the exception of acetaminophen, nonnarcotic analgesics are also useful to reduce inflammation (Table 11.2).

Parenteral Opioid Analgesia

Continuous Intravenous Infusions

The advantages of continuous infusion include easy titratability and the lack of need for cooperation (Table 11.3). The disadvantages include the potential for respiratory depression and other opioid-related side effects. Close monitoring is imperative.

TABLE 11.2. *Non-narcotic analgesics for the pediatric patient*

Oral agents	Dosages	Comments
Acetaminophen	10–15 mg/kg/dose q 4 hr PO	Maximum 2,600 mg/24 hr or 120 mg/kg/day
	10–20 mg/kg/dose q 4 hr PR*	Inconsistent rectal absorption Nephropathy and hepatotoxicity not seen with short-term use
Aspirin	10–20 mg/kg/dose q 4 hr PO	Associated with Reye's syndrome Side effects include gastritis and platelet dysfunction
Choline-magnesium salicylate (Trilisate)	10–15 mg/kg/dose q 6–8 hr PO	Questionable association with Reye's syndrome Minimal effect on platelet dysfunction or gastric lining Limited experience in young children
Ibuprofen (Motrin)	4–10 mg/kg/dose q 6–8 hr PO	May cause gastritis and platelet dysfunction Nephrotoxicity and hepatotoxicity can occur with chronic use
Naprosyn (Naproxen)	5–7 mg/kg/dose q 8–12 hr PO	As with ibuprofen
Tolectin (Tolmetin)	5–7 mg/kg/dose q 6–8 hr PO	As with ibuprofen

Reproduced from ref. 31, with permission.

PCA

Patients must be of the age to understand the concept of self-administration. This concept can be understood by most children by age 4–5 years. Thus, under age 4–5, this modality is not recommended (22,23). The initial starting PCA bolus dose is 0.01 mg/kg of morphine with a 6–10 min lockout interval. The use of basal infusions in this population is controversial. Arguments against basal infusions in pediatric patients include opioid tolerance, the increased incidence of side effects, and a reduction in the inherent safety of PCA. Others believe that basal infusions provide more adequate analgesia. The recommended dose, if utilized, is one-half to 1 PCA bolus dose.

Methadone

Methadone provides excellent analgesia for the pediatric patient.
After the initial 24 hr, maintain with a q 12 hr regimen around the clock unless the child is somnolent. See Table 11.3 for dosage guidelines.

Regional Analgesia

Use of regional analgesia (a) is limited by the expertise of the anesthesiologist; (b) employed only when consent is obtained from the parents; and (c) utilized only when skilled personnel are available to handle any complications that arise, especially when opioids are utilized (24).

Caudal Analgesia

Caudal analgesia is a useful adjunct to intraoperative anesthesia as well as for postoperative analgesia in children undergoing surgery below the level of the diaphragm (25,26). The procedure is easy to perform and has a long history of safe and efficacious use. See Table 11.4 for dosage guidelines.

Subarachnoid Opioids

Subarachnoid opioids provide excellent analgesia. Monitoring is imperative, as delayed respiratory depression is possible. The recommended does of morphine is 0.013–0.02 mg/kg (Table 11.4).

Epidural Opioids

Epidural opioids are utilized in patients usually over 2 years of age. Pain associated with lower extremity and low abdominal procedures is almost

TABLE 11.3. *Parenteral opioid analgesia for the pediatric patient*

Drug/technique	Initial loading dose	Maintenance	Weaning	Advantages	Disadvantages
Methadone	IV: 0.1 mg/kg in saline over 20 min: may repeat loading dose in 3 hr SC: 0.2 mg/kg	For IV, sliding scale, doses given q 4–6 hr (*not* prn) unless patient is somnolent or shows signs of toxicity as follows: Mild pain: 0.03 mg/kg in saline over 20 min Moderate pain: 0.05 mg/kg in saline over 20 min Severe pain: 0.07 mg/kg in saline over 20 min For SQ: 0.1 mg/kg q 4–8 hr unless somnolent	As methadone accumulates, dosing frequency is decreased to q 6 hr, then q 8 hr and q 12 hr as tolerated. In short courses of therapy, drug may be discontinued abruptly and will "self-wean" because of the long half-life.	Long half-life (infrequent dosing, self-weaning) Less euphoria and dysphoria than with other narcotics	Potent respiratory depressant Difficult to titrate because of prolonged time to onset
Morphine/PCA	Postoperative pain: 0.05–0.1 mg/kg IV (optional, based on narcotics received intraoperatively) Sickle cell crisis: 0.10–0.15 mg/kg IV	Postoperative pain: Total hourly dose: 0.05–0.1 mg/kg/hr Optional background infusion: ¼–⅓ of total hourly dose PCA bolus: remaining hourly dose divided into equal doses at 6–15 min intervals			

Drug	Loading dose	Infusion rate	Dosing notes	Advantages	Disadvantages
			Sickle cell crisis: Total hourly dose: As for postoperative pain Background infusion 2/3–3/4 of total hourly dose PCA bolus: As for postoperative pain [Promethazine (2–5 mg) may be added to 30 ml of morphine if needed for nausea and vomiting.]	Less respiratory depression seen High patient satisfaction Many patients "self-wean" by decreasing dosage frequency	Requires specialized equipment and training Requires patient participation and cooperation
Continuous infusion morphine	0.05–0.1 mg/kg IV	0.05–0.06 mg/kg/hr	As for morphine PCA	Patient cooperation and participation not required Easy to titrate to effect	Potential for respiratory depression Increased incidence of side effects (nausea, vomiting, constipation) Frequent nursing and medical observation required
Fentanyl	1–1.5 µg/kg IV	2–4 µg/kg/hr	As for morphine PCA	As for continuous infusion morphine	As for continuous infusion morphine

Reproduced from ref. 31, with permission.

completely blocked with continuous fentanyl or fentanyl-bupivacaine infusions. Continuous infusions of morphine and hydromorphone are recommended for upper abdominal and thoracic surgery. Opioid side effects include respiratory depression, pruritus and urinary retention. Pediatric patients treated with epidural opioids should be monitored continuously by trained personnel and pulse oximetry or apnea monitoring should be utilized. See Table 11.4 for dosage guidelines. Epidural bolus doses are (a) morphine, 0.05 mg/kg; (b) bupivacaine, no more than 3 mg/kg (will provide 4–6 hr of pain relief); and (c) with the volume of injectate calculated as 0.05 cc/kg/segment (include five sacral and five lumbar segments and however many thoracic segments need to be included in coverage).

Epidural infusions are as follows: (a) lower abdominal and lower extremity surgery—bupivacaine 0.1% with fentanyl 2 μg/cc at 0.3–0.5 cc/kg/hr, and bupivacaine 0.1% with morphine 0.1 mg/cc at 0.1 cc/kg/hr; (b) thoracic and upper abdominal surgery—bupivacaine 0.1% with morphine 0.1 mg/cc at 0.1 cc/kg/hr, and bupivacaine 0.1% with dilaudid 10 μg/cc at 0.3 cc/kg/hr.

Combination solutions of opioids and local anesthetics allow lower concentrations and thus lower doses of both agents to be utilized. As the child's pain subsides, one may decrease the rate of infusion or change to bupivacaine 0.1% or administer only the opioid. Such changes should be discussed with the Pediatric Pain Attending before it is performed.

Children will get quite distressed if they develop a sensory or motor block. This is not common with bupivacaine 0.1%. However, if this occurs, the local anesthetic should be eliminated from or decreased in the epidural solution.

Interpleural Analgesia

In children, effective and long-lasting pain relief has been obtained using intrapleural analgesia for postthoracotomy or upper abdominal surgical pain and pain from multiple rib fractures. McIlvaine (27) used an infusion of bupivacaine 0.25% with epinephrine 1:200,000 at the rate of 0.5 ml/kg/hr with excellent analgesia for children who had thoracotomies. The safety and efficacy of this pain management modality is still being studied.

Peripheral Neural Blockade

Peripheral nerve blocks may be utilized in the pediatric population. The age and degree of cooperation determines whether the block is performed with the child awake, lightly sedated, or under general anesthesia.

Ilioinguinal/iliohypogastric blocks provide excellent postoperative pain relief following hernia repair, hydrocelectomy, or orchiopexy. Peripheral nerve blocks may be utilized in the pediatric population. The age and degree

TABLE 11.4. Regional analgesia for the pediatric patient

Mode of delivery/drug	Dosage	Volume	Comments
Intrathecal morphine	0.01–0.025 mg/kg	As small as possible; 1 ml in children under 12 yrs	High incidence of complications (about 50%) Not indicated for infants and small children
Caudal morphine	0.03–0.05 mg/kg with bupivacaine 0.25% and epinephrine 1:200,000	Sacral levels: 0.5 ml/kg or 0.05 ml/kg/segment	Respiratory depression reported with doses of 0.1 mg/kg
Epidural morphine (administered via lumbar space)	Single dose Abdominal or lower extremities: 50 µg/kg Thoracotomy: 120–150 µg/kg Infusion	0.05–0.056 ml/kg/segment	Duration 8–24 hr
	Bupivacaine 0.1% + morphine 0.1 mg/ml	0.1 ml/kg/hr	Continuous levels of analgesia achieved
Epidural fentanyl	0.5–1 µg/kg single dose	0.05 ml/kg/segment	Duration: 3–4 hr Lipid solubility may necessitate higher volume of injectate to achieve levels similar to morphine
Epidural sufentanil	0.75 µg/kg single dose	0.05 ml/kg/segment	Duration: 2 hr High lipid solubility suggests continuous infusion will be more effective for long-term analgesia

Reproduced from ref. 31, with permission.

of cooperation determines whether the block can be performed with the child awake, lightly sedated, or under general anesthesia.

Penile nerve blocks may be utilized for surgical procedures on the penis, i.e., circumcision or correction of a distal hypospadias.

Intercostal nerve blocks may be used for thoracic and upper abdominal surgical procedures, rib fractures, and, as in adults, for the diagnosis of pain syndromes.

Transcutaneous Electrical Nerve Stimulation

Although primarily used in chronic pain syndromes, postthoracotomy and cardiac surgical patients may use this as an adjuvant to opioid therapy.

Topical Anesthetics

Topical anesthetics may be utilized to anesthetize mucosal surfaces. The extent and duration of analgesia depends upon the local anesthetic, dose, and concentration administered.

SICKLE CELL CRISIS

Painful crises in a patient with sickle cell disease are intermittent, repetitive, and unpredictable with respect to timing and the location of pain. Most episodes last 4–5 days, but may be as short as hours or as long as weeks (28). There is a wide spectrum ranging from acute to chronic pain because of the variability of the pain among people with sickle cell disease (29).

PCA is highly effective in patients suffering from sickle cell crisis. Self administered dose requirements are significantly lower than amounts utilized with continuous opioid infusion therapy. Morphine is the drug of choice for sickle cell crisis. Acutely, PCA is always combined with a basal infusion. The total dose is started at 0.1–0.2 mg/kg/hr. Two-thirds of this dose is provided as a continuous infusion, with one-third made available as PCA bolus doses. Patients are seen frequently in the first 24 hr, and adjustments in dosage are made according to the patient's response. Over a period of days, the basal infusion is gradually tapered while the PCA bolus doses are maintained. Transition to long-acting oral opioids can then be made.

NSAIDs are useful adjuncts, especially where bone and joint pain predominates. Ketorolac, an intramuscular/intravenous NSAID, may significantly reduce PCA opioid requirements.

One common side effect observed with PCA in this population is nausea and vomiting. The severity of nausea may be reduced by adding small doses of promethazine 0.1 mg/kg to each 30 ml syringe of PCA morphine. Diphenhydramine and metoclopramide are also effective antiemetics.

Scopolamine and droperidol should be used with caution in patients under 18 years of age, as they may produce psychotomimetic reactions; droperidol is also associated with occulogyrocrises.

SUBSTANCE ABUSE PATIENT

Postoperative pain therapy must be provided for the substance abuse patient. PCA, spinal opioids, and other modalities may all be used, but one should be cognizant of the greater opioid requirements and potential for opioid withdrawal. The use of adjuvant drugs (e.g., methadone, librium, ativan, clonidine) is often necessary in this population. Furthermore, the use of opioid agonist-antagonists are to be avoided, as acute withdrawal can be precipitated. Spinal opioids will provide excellent analgesia, but maintenance parenteral opioid must be administered concomitantly to prevent withdrawal.

Stacey et al. (30) showed that PCA can effectively be utilized in patients with a substance abuse history. Their findings suggest that substance abuse patients require larger doses of opioids to achieve postoperative pain relief than do opioid-free patients, but their need for this additional medication is not prolonged. The increased use does not appear to reflect abuse; it reflects a combination of factors including tolerance, habituation, and the patient's coping skills. In our institution, we have also effectively utilized PCA in substance abuse patients. We have found that the majority of patients can effectively use PCA, as supported by Stacey. However, some patients, whether secondary to coping mechanisms or the lack of sedation, are not effectively managed with PCA. These patients are managed using intramuscular opioid injections combined with hydroxyzine hydrochloride.

SUMMARY

Pain intensity varies significantly depending on the surgical stimulus, thus the approach to pain management must allow for these variations. Table 11.5 summarizes the choice of pain modalities for specific surgical populations.

TABLE 11.5. Pain modality for specific surgical populations

Surgery	PCA opioid	Spinal opioid	Intrapleural analgesia	Nerve block
Gynecologic	Meperidine Hydromorphone Morphine	No clear preference	Not applicable	Not applicable
Obstetric	Hydromorphone Meperidine Morphine	Meperidine Morphine Sufentanil/fentanyl	Not applicable	Not applicable
Orthopedics	Hydromorphone Morphine Basal infusion frequently requested Consider NSAIDs as adjuvant therapy	Continuous infusion of morphine, fentanyl, sufentanil, or meperidine in combination with dilute bupivacaine	For management of rib fractures	Excellent therapy for extremity surgery alone or in combination with parenteral opioids
General surgery	Morphine hydromorphone	Morphine Lipophilic agents especially if via thoracic catheter Bolus doses or continuous infusion	Good for upper abdominal procedures	Minimal application
Urologic	Meperidine	Sufentanil/fentanyl Morphine Meperidine	Good for flank incisions	Consider block for penile surgery, intercostal block for flank incision
Vascular	No clear preferences	Morphine by bolus or intermittent bolus or continuous infusion Fentanyl/sufentanil	Not applicable	Will provide sympathectomy and improved circulation outcome with limb/digit reimplantation

REFERENCES

1. Brown JG. Systemic opioid analgesia for postoperative pain management. In: Benumof JL, Oden RV, eds. *Management of postoperative pain. Anesthesiology clinics of North America.* 1989;7:1:51.
2. Yeager MP. Outcome of pain management. In: Benumof JL, Oden RV, eds. *Management of postoperative pain. Anesthesiology Clinics of North America.* 1989;7:1:241.
3. Burns JW, Hodsman NBA, McLintock TTC, Gillies GWA, Kenny GNC, McArdle CS. The influence of patient characteristics on the requirements for postoperative analgesia. *Anaesthesia* 1989;44:2–6.
4. Belville JW, Forrest WH, Miller E, Brown BW. Influence of age on pain relief from analgesics. *JAMA* 1971;217:1835–1841.
5. White PF. Patient-controlled analgesia: an update on its use in the treatment of postoperative pain. In: Benumof JL, Oden RV, eds. *Management of postoperative pain. Anesthesiology clinics of North America.* 1989;7:1:63.
6. McCaffery M, Beebe A. *Pain—clinical manual for nursing practice.* St. Louis, MO: C.V. Mosby Co., 1989.
7. Sinatra RS, Lodge K, Sibert K, Chung KS, Chung JH, Parker A, Harrison D. A comparison of morphine, meperidine and oxymorphone as utilized in patient-controlled analgesia following cesarean delivery. *Anesthesiology* 1989;70;585–590.
8. Wittels B, Scott DT, Sinatra RS. Exogenous opioids in human breast milk and acute neonatal neurobehavior: a preliminary study. *Anesthesiology* 1990;73:864–869.
9. Deutsch EV. Postoperative analgesia with hydromorphone and meperidine. A double-blind comparison. *Anesthiol Anal* 1968;47:669–671.
10. Harrison DM, Sinatra R, Morgese L, Chung JH. Epidural narcotic and patient-controlled analgesia for post-cesarean section pain relief. *Anesthesiology* 1988;68:454–457.
11. Chadwick HS, Ross BK. Analgesia for post-cesarian delivery pain. In: Benumof JL, Oden RV, eds. *Management of postoperative pain. Anesthesiology clinics of North America.* 1989; 7:1:133.
12. White PF. Patient-controlled analgesia: A new approach to the management of postoperative pain. *Semin Anesth* 1985;4:255–266.
13. Harris SN, Sevarino FB, Silverman DG, Preble L, Sinatra RS. Prophylactic transdermal scopolamine for patients using patient controlled analgesia (PCA). *Anesthesiology* 1989; 71:3A690.
14. Freilich JD, Sinatra RS, Jankelovitz ER, Preble L, Sevarino FB, Silverman DG. Morphine plus promethazine for patient controlled analgesia. *Anesth Analg* 1990;70:S373.
15. Greenblatt DJ, Sellers EM, Shader RI. Medical intelligence. *N Engl J Med* 1982;306: 1081–1088.
16. Tuman KJ, McCarthy RJ, Ivankovich AD. Pain control in the postoperative cardiac surgery patient. *Hosp Formul* 1988;23:580–595.
17. El-Baz NMI, Faber LP, Jensik RJ. Continuous epidural infusion of morphine for treatment of pain after thoracic surgery: a new technique. *Anesth Analg* 1984;63:757–764.
18. Cullen ML, Staren ED, El-Ganzouri A, Logas WG, Ivankovich AD, Economou SG. Continuous epidural infusion for analgesia after major abdominal operations: a randomized, prospective, double-blind study. *Surgery* 1985;98:718–728.
19. Fischer RL, Lubenow TR, Liceaga A, McCarthy RJ, Ivankovich AD. Comparison of continuous epidural infusion of fentanyl-bupivacaine and morphine-bupivacaine in management of postoperative pain. *Anesth Analg* 1988;67:559–563.
20. Tomlin PJ. After-care following abdominal vascular surgery. In: Wright J, ed. *Anaesthesia for vascular surgery.* London: Butterworth and Co., 1988:194–200.
21. Raggi R, Dardik HD, Mauro AL. Continuous epidural anesthesia and postoperative epidural narcotics in vascular surgery. *Am J Surg* 1987;154:192–197.
22. Rodgers BM, Webb CJ, Stergios D, Newman BM. Patient-controlled analgesia in pediatric surgery. *J Pediatr Surg* 1988;23:259–262.
23. Webb CJ, Stergios DA, Rodgers BM. Patient-controlled analgesia as postoperative pain treatment for children. *J Pediatr Nurs* 1989;4:162–171.
24. Yaster M, Maxwell LG. Pediatric regional anesthesia. *Anesthesiology* 1989;70:324–338.

25. Fell D, Derrington MC, Taylor E, Wandless JG. Paediatric postoperative analgesia: a comparison between caudal block and wound infiltration of local anaesthetic. *Anaesthesia* 1988;43:107–110.
26. McGown RG. Caudal analgesia in children. Five hundred cases for procedures below the diaphragm. *Anaesthesia* 1982;37:806–818.
27. McIlvaine WB, Knox RF, Fennessey PV, Goldstein M. Continuous infusion of bupivacaine via intrapleural catheter for analgesia after thoracotomy in children. *Anesthesiology* 1988;69:261–264.
28. Berde CB, Sethna NF, DeJesus JM, Yemen TA, Mandell J. Continuous epidural bupivacaine-fentanyl infusions in children undergoing urologic surgery. *Anesth Analg* 1990;70: S1–S450.
29. Morrison RA, Vedro DA. Pain management in the child with sickle cell disease. *Pediatr Nurs* 1989;15:6:595–599.
30. Stacey BR, Brody MC, Burke DF. Patients with a substance abuse history can effectively use PCA. *Anesthesiology* 1990;73:A759.
31. Bell C, Hughes CW, Oh TH. In: Gay SM (ed) *The Pediatric Anesthesia Handbook,* St. Louis, Mosby–Year Book, Inc., 1991.

SUGGESTED READINGS

Stacey BR, Brody MC, Burke DF. Patients with a substance abuse history can effectively use PCA. *Anesthesiology* 1990;73:A759.
Harrison DM, Sinatra R, Morgese L, Chung JH. Epidural narcotic and patient-controlled analgesia for post-cesarean section pain relief. *Anesthesiology* 1988;68:454–457.
Loper KA, Rady LB. Epidural morphine after anterior cruciate ligament repair: a comparison with patient-controlled intravenous morphine. *Anesth Analg* 1989;68:350–352.
Owen H, Kluger MT, Plummer JL. Variables of patient-controlled analgesia 4: the relevance of bolus dose size to supplement a background infusion. *Anaesthesia* 1990;45:619–622.
Stein C, Comisel K, Yassouridis A, Herz A, Peter K. Intra-articular morphine produces analgesia following arthroscopic knee surgery. *Anesthesiology* 1990;73:A765.

12

Illustrative Cases

CASE 1

A 35-year-old, 130-kg woman with a history of severe asthma, morbid obesity, and chronic back pain with neurological deficit secondary to disc herniation, presented for a T11–T12 anterior spinal discectomy and fusion. Her anesthetic included isoflurane, vecuronium, and fentanyl (a total of 3,000 μg). The surgeon is concerned about her respiratory problems as related to her postoperative pain management.

Discussion

Postoperatively, the patient is at risk for atelectasis secondary to inactivity and pain, and also opioid induced respiratory depression. Pain relief could be optimized with IV patient controlled analgesia (IV-PCA). The drug of choice in this patient is hydromorphone which is 6–8 times more potent than morphine, and provides effective relief of periosteal pain. Further, hydromorphone is more efficacious than meperidine and is less likely to cause histamine release as seen with morphine. This is important in light of the history of asthma. The incremental dose of hydromorphone should be 0.1–0.25 mg with a lockout of 6–8 min. A basal infusion of 0.1–0.25 mg/hr may be considered during the first 24 hr, if clinically indicated.

Analgesia may be supplemented with a loading dose of ketorolac 60 mg IM, followed by 30 mg every 6 hr. Because of the additive analgesic effects, a basal infusion of hydromorphone is usually not required when ketorolac is utilized. Small doses of diazepam (5–10 mg q 6–8 hr) or other muscle relaxants may be administered should muscle spasms occur. Since these adjuvant drugs may potentiate the sedative effects of the opioid, the PCA dose, lockout interval, and basal infusion should be adjusted downward when employing these agents. Furthermore, since this patient is morbidly obese, has a history of asthma, and has received a large dose of fentanyl intra-

195

operatively, she is at increased risk for respiratory compromise. This patient should be monitored by pulse oximetry for the first 12–24 hr, and supplemental oxygen should be administered if indicated.

CASE 2

An otherwise healthy 16-year-old is status postthoracotomy for a nonmalignant cyst and had an epidural catheter placed at the L3–4 interspace for postoperative pain management. An overnight stay in the Pediatric Intensive Care Unit is planned. An infusion of morphine (50 μg/ml) at a rate of 15–20 ml/hr is started. Four hours later, the patient is complaining of pain.

Discussion

Young vigorous patients recovering from thoracic surgery often present difficult acute pain management problems. Opioids administered via lumbar epidural catheters provide less effective analgesia than when given through catheters placed at thoracic levels. Nevertheless, morphine is the drug of choice, as it will ascend in the CSF from a lumbar administered site to reach thoracic spinal sites. Morphine may be administered as either an intermittent bolus of 5–10 mg every 12–20 hr in a volume of 10–20 ml of normal saline diluent, or as a continuous infusion at a maximum rate of no more than 1 mg/hr. This patient is presently at the maximum infusion rate.

As the patient is complaining of pain, the catheter should first be tested to ensure proper positioning. Test the catheter with 3–5 ml of 1.5% lidocaine with epinephrine 1:200,000. If an anesthetic level is detected, we first administer 50–100 μg fentanyl in 10–20 ml normal saline epidurally to gain immediate control of the pain. A dilute concentration of bupivacaine (0.5–0.1%) may then be added to the opioid infusion. Dilute solutions rarely block sympathetic or motor fibers, yet will synergize the analgesic effect of the opioid, thereby improving pain relief. If the catheter is properly positioned but pain relief is still not optimal, other analgesic adjuncts should be considered: Small doses of intravenous morphine (1–2 mg IV) or diazepam (1–2 mg IV) will provide anxiolysis and may also provide supraspinal analgesia. Often patients are actually comfortable but are very alert and anxious. Thus, careful titration of anxiolytics is important. Monitoring should include continuous pulse oximetry, EKG and frequent vital signs. Arterial blood gases should be obtained as indicated.

CASE 3

A 43-year-old man is status postnephrectomy. His medical history is significant for alcohol abuse. A lumbar epidural catheter has been placed intraoperatively for postoperative pain management. An infusion of morphine (50 μg/mg/ml) and bupivacaine (0.1 mg/ml) was instituted at a rate of 12 ml/hr.

Discussion

Patients with histories of substance abuse are difficult to manage in the postoperative period, even when highly effective analgesia is provided. The combination of morphine and bupivacaine usually provides excellent pain relief. However, even minor discomfort may agitate such patients. Should this occur, intravenous diazepam, lorazepam or morphine may be titrated to decrease anxiety and supplement analgesia. Lorazepam or chlordiazepoxide should be administered to attenuate or prevent alcohol withdrawal symptoms, especially if the patient has been drinking heavily prior to the surgical procedure. If the patient abuses opioids, morphine or methadone should be administered intravenously, as the small amount of morphine administered epidurally may not prevent central opioid withdrawal. Clonidine, either administered orally or transdermally, has also been shown to reduce the symptoms of withdrawal in substance abuse patients.

CASE 4

A 70-year-old man is recovering from radical cystectomy performed under spinal anesthesia. He was premedicated with diazepam 10 mg orally. As part of the spinal anesthetic, the patient receiving intrathecal morphine 0.8 mg (1.6 ml). He is pain free following the resolution of the sensory motor blockade.

Discussion

Patients at the extremes of age are acutely sensitive to the sedative and respiratory effects of spinal opioids. This sensitivity may be heightened by the concomitant use of benzodiazepines, scopolamine, parenteral opioids, or other sedatives administered pre- or intraoperatively. The dose and volume of morphine administered was relatively high for a patient of this age. If his respiratory rate and oxygen saturation should decrease or should he become somnolent, a naloxone infusion 0.5–1 μg/kg/hr should be started. (This could be administered prophylactically.) As this patient is pain free, the degree of CNS depression associated with the diazepam premedication may become profound. Small amounts of physostigmine, (0.5–2 mg) given intravenously in divided doses, may reverse an excessive level of sedation should it occur. This patient should be observed for 24 hr in an intensive care setting with cardiac monitor or pulse oximetry.

CASE 5

A 23-year-old woman, gravida 1, para 1, underwent cesarean delivery, under epidural anesthesia using 2% lidocaine and 3% chloroprocaine. She received 5 mg of epidural morphine 4 hr earlier and is now complaining of severe pruritus and abdominal discomfort.

Discussion

Chloroprocaine has been shown to antagonize spinal analgesia provided by epidural opioids. The low PH of chloroprocaine may influence the uptake of morphine. Thus, it might be best to avoid spinal opioids in patients receiving chloroprocaine or administer them after dissipation of chloroprocaine's effects.

Pruritus occurs in over 70% of obstetrical patients who receive spinally administered morphine. It may be treated with diphenhydramine (12.5–50 mg IV, IM, or PO) or with small doses of naloxone (40 μg IV followed by a 0.5–1-μg/kg/hr infusion) in patients who are otherwise pain free. Given this patient's inadequate analgesia, naloxone would not be appropriate. Small amounts of nalbuphine, a mixed opioid agonist/antagonist (5 mg IV followed by 10 mg/L of IV fluid), would offer benefits of additive analgesia, while decreasing the intensity of pruritus. Analgesia may be supplemented with IV-PCA, using a decreased dose of meperidine (5–10 mg every 10–15 min). If a nonopioid analgesic is preferred, ketorolac 15–30 mg IV or IM q 6 hr can be used.

CASE 6

A 62-year-old woman with a history of hypertension treated with propranolol is receiving PCA therapy (morphine 1 mg q 8 min) following her hysterectomy. She has severe nausea and vomiting. Intraoperatively she received fentanyl (500 mcg), nitrous oxide, and isoflurane.

Discussion

Nausea is the most common side effect associated with IV-PCA opioid therapy, and its incidence is especially high following pelvic surgery. The combination of pelvic manipulation, visceral ligation, and beta-blockade may lead to increased vagal tone with associated nausea and vomiting. Opioids further exacerbate the problem by increasing vagal tone and by directly effecting the brainstem emesis center. Transdermal scopolamine will effectively reduce both the incidence and severity of nausea. However, its peak effect may not be appreciated for at least four hours following application. Patients over 60 years of age may experience psychological effects from this medication. Thus, in this patient, we usually administer droperidol 0.625–1.25 mg IV or metoclopramide 5–10 mg IV to treat nausea. Lowering the PCA morphine dose from 1 mg every 8 min to 0.7 or 0.8 mg every 6 min may reduce peak morphine levels and associated nausea. Switching from morphine to meperidine, a drug that has less vagal effects, may also decrease her nausea. Nausea and vomiting occurring the first or second postoperative day may be secondary to an ileus, a bowel obstruction, or another surgical problem, and should be discussed with the surgeon.

CASE 7

A 39-year-old man is undergoing abdominoplasty. He has a history of alcohol and drug abuse, but denies use of these substances for the past 3 years. He requested not to be given any opiates. The surgeon has consulted the APS for postoperative pain management.

Discussion

Patients with histories of substance abuse often fear opioid administration in the postsurgical period, as they are concerned about re-addiction. Epidural analgesia is an excellent option in this situation as it provides superior analgesia with minimal dose requirements and central opioid effects (i.e., sedation, euphoria, etc.). In this patient, epidural (and intrathecal) opioids offer an ideal analgesic choice with respect to the surgical site as well. Pulmonary function is markedly impaired postoperatively in obese patients or in patients who have had lengthy upper abdominal surgery. Epidural morphine has been shown to preserve forced vital capacity (FVC) to a greater degree than parenteral opioids. Thus, this patient can obtain superior pain control, while avoiding the central opioid effects. If epidural analgesia is not feasible, ketorolac may be used to lower the total opioid requirements.

If the patient is on a methadone maintenance program and is receiving methadone preoperatively, the maintenance dose must be given postoperatively to avoid withdrawal symptoms. Opioid agonist/antagonists should also be avoided in this patient population.

CASE 8

A 41-year-old man, with a history of multiple drug allergies and a previously severe reaction to morphine, developed total body urticaria and bronchospasm following administration of meperidine during a cholecystectomy. Postoperatively, the patient is stable, but has severe incisional pain.

Discussion

Both morphine and to a lesser extent meperidine, cause mast cell degranulation and histamine release. In contrast, the more potent-lipophilic opioids fentanyl and sufentanil rarely cause histamine release. This patient should be treated with histamine type 1 and type 2 blocking drugs during the first 24 hr postoperatively. Analgesic requirements can be met, utilizing IV-PCA fentanyl or sufentanil. Fentanyl 10–20 μg with a lockout interval of 6 min and a basal infusion of 10–20 μg/hr should be employed for the first 12 hr following surgery. Doses can be adjusted as needed for pain relief. The patient may also be a candidate for intrathecal opioids or interpleural analgesia. Both alternatives would provide excellent postoperative analgesia. Ketorolac (intramuscular/intravenous) is another option for pain management.

CASE 9

A 16-year-old woman with sickle beta-thalassemia disease presents in painful crisis.

Discussion

Painful crises in sickle cell disease are believed to be caused by ischemia tissue injury resulting from obstruction of blood flow by sickled erythrocytes. In general, there are three essential needs in the management of a crisis: hydration, adequate analgesia, and treatment of the precipitating factors (e.g., infection, depression, etc.).

The goal of analgesic therapy is to provide optimal pain management. The choice of analgesic is based on potency, duration, and side effects. PCA morphine with a basal infusion is ideal in this patient population, as it maintains a steady serum drug level, improves the management of pain, and decreases anxiety by providing the patient with "control of his pain management." We usually start with a total dose of 0.1–0.2 mg/kg/hr; the basal infusion is two-thirds of the total hourly dose; the PCA increment is the remaining one-third. PCA demerol in equianalgesic doses is employed in patients in which sickle cell crisis is superimposed upon cholecystitis/cholelithiasis. The crisis usually lasts approximately 48–72 hr, at which time the basal infusion is tapered daily by 10% until usage is minimal (4–7 days). The addition of a NSAID to the opioid therapy may improve analgesia and decrease opioid requirements. However, caution is advised in utilizing NSAIDs in sickle cell patients with renal dysfunction.

CASE 10

A 25-year-old man, with a history of lymphoma, has undergone retroperitoneal and periaortic node biopsies. He is referred to the APS for management of severe postsurgical pain. IV-PCA with morphine (1.0 mg every 6 min, plus a basal infusion of 0.5 mg/hr), was initiated. The patient received 111 mg of morphine during a 36-hr period (approximately 3 mg/hr). Approximately 30 min after a visit from family members and friends, the patient was found unresponsive with a temperature of 104°F and a respiratory rate of 10–12. Arterial blood gas (ABG) indicated acidosis (pH 7.16, PCO_2 63, PO_2 60,). He was given 1,200 mcg of naloxone by the surgical house officer. The patient's respiratory rate increased to 30 breaths/min. The patient remained sedated for the next 24 hr but had a complete and uncomplicated recovery.

Discussion

A patient's underlying disease, as well as events occurring in the postsurgical period, can markedly influence sensitivity and response to opioids. This patient had been doing well, but developed sepsis on the second postoperative day. Sepsis of this magnitude, and the lymphoma itself, may have affected the blood brain barrier, allowing greater penetration of morphine into the CNS. Plasma morphine levels were found to be within normal range. Thus, it is important to adjust therapy based on the patient's medical condition. Further, given the events that occurred here, it is important to have a protocol to address adverse events related to acute pain therapies. Appendix 1.5 outlines the Adverse Event Protocol used by the APS at Yale–New Haven Hospital/Yale University.

Appendix 2.1: Drugs and Indications for
Use in Acute Pain Management

Indications and dosages are suggested only. Not all indications discussed are
FDA approved. Please consult references before using medications with
which you are not familiar.

I. ANTIEMETICS
   A. **Benzquinamide hydrochloride (Emete-Con):** Benzquinamide is a
      short-acting benquinoline derivative that inhibits stimuli at the
      chemoreceptor trigger zone.
      1. Side effects
         a. Drowsiness is the most common adverse reaction.
         b. Mild anticholinergic effects have occurred.
         c. Direct relaxation of vascular smooth muscle may result
            in decreased peripheral vascular resistance (PVR) and
            hypotension. Reflex sympathetic compensation in-
            creases norepinephrine, thus increasing HR, and CO,
            and may cause sudden increase in blood pressure and
            dysrhythmia, *particularly if given rapidly IV.*
      2. Nursing considerations
         a. Overdosage may be manifested as either a central
            anticholinergic syndrome 2° to its anticholinergic
            properties (responsive to physostigmine), or dys-
            tonic extrapyramidine reactions (exacerbated by
            physostigmine).
         b. Administration to patient with moderate to severe
            hypertension or severe cardiovascular disease is ques-
            tionable.
      3. Dosage and administration
         a. Intramuscular: 0.5–1.0 mg/kg to a maximum of 50
            mg—may repeat in 1 hr, then every 3–4 hr as necessary
         b. Intravenous: 0.2–0.4 mg/kg to a maximum of 25 mg
            administered *slowly over 3–5-min period to avoid
            hypertension and dysrhythmia. Give subsequent doses
            IM.*
         c. Intramuscular administration is preferred.
      4. Pharmacokinetics
         a. Onset is usually within 15 min
         b. Elimination half-time: 40 min
         c. 58% plasma bound
         d. Metabolized in the liver
   B. **Droperidol (Inapsine):** Droperidol is a butyrophenone which
      structurally resembles phenothiazines (Compazine, Thorazine)
      and evokes similar pharmacologic effects. It acts postsynapti-
      cally to decrease the neurotransmitter function of dopamine; its

antiemetic effect is through inhibition of these dopaminergic receptors in the chemoreceptor trigger zone of the medulla.

1. Side effects
   a. Can cause mild hypotension secondary to peripheral alpha-adrenergic antagonism. This becomes significant only in the setting of hypovolemia.
   b. As a dopamine agonist, droperidol may occasionally evoke extrapyramidal reactions.
   c. Dysphoria
   d. Sedation
   e. Exaggerates the respiratory depressant effects of narcotics and the sedative effects of CNS depressants.
2. Nursing considerations
   a. The manifestations of droperidol overdosage are an extension of its pharmacologic actions, i.e., hypotension, tachycardia, and sedation.
3. Dosage and administration
   a. 1.25–2.5 mg intravenously prior to emergence from anesthesia decreases postoperative nausea and vomiting.
   b. Effective postoperative dose for antiemetic effects is 0.25–0.625 mg (0.1–0.25 ml) IV every 4 hr as needed.
4. Pharmacokinetics
   a. Onset of action is 3–10 min following IV or IM administration. Peak 30 min.
   b. Elimination half-time of 150 μg/kg is 104 min.
   c. Metabolized by the liver with maximal excretion of metabolites with 24 hr.
   d. Total body clearance of 14.1 ml kg^{-1} (similar to hepatic blood flow)

C. **Metoclopramide hydrochloride (Reglan):** Metoclopramide is a dopamine antagonist which increases the strength of contractions of the gastric antrum and speeds gastric emptying. It also increases lower esophageal sphincter tone by 10–20 cm H_2O. Metoclopramide antagonizes dopamine receptors in the CNS and may produce extrapyramidal symptoms.

1. Side effects
   a. Side effects are infrequent and have not been observed after single doses of metoclopramide. They include sedation, akinesia, and extrapyramidal reactions.
2. Nursing considerations
   a. If IV injection is too rapid, a transient but intense feeling of anxiety and restlessness may occur.

3. Dosage and administration
   a. For treatment of nausea and vomiting: 10–20 mg IV over 1–5 min
   b. For nausea prophylaxis: 10–20 mg PO/IV every 4–6 hr
   c. PO: 10 mg before meals
4. Pharmacokinetics
   a. Rapidly absorbed after oral administration, about 50–70% with total bioavailability.
   b. Onset time 1–3 min following an IV dose; 10–15 min following IM dose; 30–60 min following a PO dose.
   c. Metoclopramide is eliminated unchanged (approximately 30%) or conjugated by the kidney in 2–4 hr.
   d. Half-life is approximately 3–6 hr.
   e. Impaired renal function prolongs the elimination half-time, as metoclopramide is primarily excreted in the urine.

D. **Prochloroperazine (Compazine):** Prochloroperazine is a phenothiazine derivative of the piperazine group. It exerts an antiemetic effect by antagonizing dopaminergic receptors in the chemoreceptor trigger zone in the medulla. It may exaggerate the respiratory depressant and sedative effects of narcotics and potentiate the analgesic effects. Prochloroperazine is available in 13 dosage forms and strengths for oral, rectal and parenteral administration.
   1. Side effects
      a. See side effects of droperidol
      b. Dystonia
      c. Anticholinergic effects including blurred vision, decreased salivation
      d. Direct cardiac depression
      e. Contraindications: glaucoma; use with caution in pediatrics.
   2. Nursing considerations
      a. The antiemetic action of prochloroperazine may mask the signs and symptoms of overdosage from other drugs.
   3. Dosage and administration
      a. Oral: 5–10 mg q 6–8 hr; *or* Spansule capsule: one 15 mg sustained release capsule every morning; or 10 mg q 12 hr—do not crush capsules.
      b. Rectal: 25 mg q 12 hr
      c. Intramuscular: 5–10 mg q 3–4 hr. Total dose should not exceed 40 mg in one 24–hr period.
      d. Intravenous: 5–10 mg. May repeat once if necessary.

Rate of administration should not exceed 5 mg/ml/min. Do not use bolus injection as it may cause hypotension.

  e. Subcutaneous administration is not advisable because of local irritation and may cause tissue necrosis.

  f. Children over the age of 2 years: PO or rectal: 9.1–13.2 kg, 2.5 mg 1 or 2 times daily; 13.6–17.7 kg, 2.5 mg 2 or 3 times daily; 18.2–38.6 kg, 2.5 mg 3 times daily or 5 mg twice daily.

  g. Intramuscular: 0.132 mg/kg. Duration of action may be 12 hr.

4. Pharmacokinetics

  a. Onset time: 15 min following IV dose

  b. Elimination half-time: 10–20 hr

  c. Metabolism primarily by oxidation and conjugation in the liver

  d. Metabolites eliminated in the urine

E. **Promethazine hydrochloride (Phenergan):** Promethazine is a phenothiazine derivative with antiemetic effects similar to prochlorperizine. It also posseses antihistamine effects.

1. Side effects

  a. See prochloroperizine

  b. Phenergan contains sodium metabisulfite, which may cause allergic reactions in susceptible individuals.

2. Nursing considerations

  a. See prochloroperizine

  b. Intra-arterial injection causes vasospasm and may result in gangrene of the affected extremity.

  c. Subcutaneous injection may cause tissue necrosis.

3. Dosage and administration

  a. As an adjunct to intramuscular narcotic pain medication for nausea prophylaxis, 25–50 mg q 4 hr IM

  b. For treatment of nausea and vomiting, 12.5–25 mg q 4 hr, either IM, IV, orally, or per rectum.

  c. May be used in combination with morphine or meperidine PCA: add 25 mg to a 30 mg morphine or 300 mg meperidine syringe.

  d. For children under 12 years of age, do not exceed more than one-half the adult dose.

  e. Do not give intra-arterial or SQ as it may cause irritation and/or necrosis.

4. Pharmacokinetics

  a. Onset of action within 15–60 min following oral dose.

  b. Duration of 4 to 6 hr.

  c. Metabolized by the liver.

F. **Transdermal scopolamine:** Transdermal scopolamine is a belladonna alkaloid used in the prevention of labrynthine-induced nausea and vomiting (motion sickness). It provides sustained therapeutic plasma levels for treatment and prophylaxis of nausea and vomiting. Scopolamine antagonizes cholinergic postganglionic muscarinic receptors. Its antiemetic effect is believed to be secondary to inhibition of transmission from the vestibular apparatus to the medulla, thereby diminishing the vomiting reflex.

1. Side effects
    a. Sedation/restlessness/disorientation/confusion
    b. Decreased salivation (dry mouth)
    c. Mydriasis
    d. Cycloplegia (blurred vision)
    e. Urinary retention
2. Nursing considerations
    a. Hands should be thoroughly washed with soap and water immediately after handling the disc, as mydriasis and cycloplegia can occur if the drug comes into contact with the eyes.
    b. Only one patch should be on the patient at a time.
    c. Each patch is active for 3 days.
    d. Use with caution in patients with glaucoma, urinary bladder neck obstruction.
    e. Use with caution in patients over 60 and under 18 years of age.
    f. Discontinue the patch if blurred vision or dizziness occurs.
3. Dosage and administration
    a. Each transdermal scopolamine patch releases scopolamine at a controlled, constant rate, delivering a total of 0.5 mg over a 3-day period (72 hr). It is applied over the mastoid area.
    b. For nausea prophylaxis apply patch 2–4 hours prior to emergence for anesthesia
4. Pharmacokinetics
    a. Scopolamine is almost entirely hydrolyzed to an inactive metabolite, only about 10% is excreted unchanged in the urine.
G. **Trimethobenzamide hydrochloride (Tigan):** Trimethobenzamide hydrochloride is an antihistamine that exerts an antiemetic effect by inhibiting stimuli at the chemoreceptor trigger zone in the medulla. It is not as effective as phenothiazines in treating postoperative nausea.

1. Side effects
   a. Extrapyramidal reactions
   b. Hypotension, blood dyscrasias, blurring of vision, coma, convulsions, depression, diarrhea, disorientation, dizziness, drowsiness, headache, jaundice, muscle cramps, and opisthotonos have also been reported.
2. Nursing considerations
   a. With the exception of sedation, side effects are not common.
3. Dosage and administration
   a. Oral: 250 mg capsule q 6–8 hr children (13.6–40.9 kg), 100–200 mg, 3 or 4 times daily
   b. Rectal Suppositories: 200 mg q 6–8 hr; these contain benzocaine and thus should not be used in patients with known sensitivities to this or similar local anesthetics
   c. Intramuscular: 200 mg q 6–8 hr
   d. Intravenous or subcutaneous administration not recommended
4. Pharmacokinetics
   a. Metabolized in the liver

H. **Hydroxyzine (Vistaril):** Hydroxyzine is a piperazine antihistamine. In addition to antiemetic effects, it has antispasmodic properties.
   1. Side Effects
      a. Potentiates CNS depressants.
   2. Nursing considerations
      a. May cause drowsiness
      b. May cause dry mouth
   3. Dosage and administration
      a. Oral: 50–100 mg 4 times daily. Children over 6, 50–100 mg daily; children under 6, 50 mg daily.
      b. Intramuscular: 25–100 mg 4–6 times daily. Children, 1.1 mg/kg.
   4. Pharmacokinetics
      a. Orally—rapidly absorbed from GI tract clinical effects are usually seen within 15–30 min.
      b. Mean elimination half-life is 3 hr.
      c. Metabolized by the liver.

II. OPIOID AGONISTS/AGONIST–ANTAGONISTS/ANTAGONIST: Opioids interact with specific receptors in the CNS which are usually the site of action of endorphin. There are at least four different types of opioid receptors: mu, delta, kappa, and sigma (see Table 2.1).

TABLE 2.1. *Opioid receptors*

Receptor type	Effect
Mu	Supraspinal analgesia
	Spinal
	Respiratory depression
	Euphoria
	Miosis
Delta	Supraspinal analgesia
	Euphoria
	Respiratory depression
	Bradycardia
Kappa	Spinal analgesia
	Respiratory depression
	Miosis
	Sedation
Sigma	Dysphoria
	Hallucination
	Mydriasis

A. **Opioid agonists:**
   Opioid agonist analgesics are indicated for the relief of moderate to severe pain. All have abuse potential. Rapid IV injection increases the incidence of adverse reactions. Use caution when administering SQ or IM in hypothermic patients, as impaired perfusion may prevent complete absorption. In general, the shorter the onset and duration of action of the opiate, the greater the intensity and rapidity of onset. Therapeutic doses of opioids may decrease respiratory drive while simultaneously increasing airway resistance. Therefore, opioids should be used with caution in patients with respiratory conditions. The sedative affects of antihistamines, phenothiazines, barbiturates, tranquilizers, sedative-hypnotics, tricyclic antidepressants, and other CNS depressants may be potentiated with concomitant use of opioids.
   1. **Morphine:** Morphine is the prototype opioid agonist, against which all other opioids are compared. It is derived from opium, although it can also be synthesized.
      a. Side effects
         i. Dose-related depression of respiration
         ii. Reduced peripheral vascular resistance
         iii. Urinary retention
         iv. Bronchospasm secondary to histamine release
         v. Pruritus

    b. Nursing considerations
- i. Respiratory depression is dose-related and responds to naloxone
- ii. Pruritus may be treated by an antihistamine or naloxone
- iii. Contraindications: allergy to morphine; reactive airway disease

    c. Dosage and administration
- i. Intramuscular/subcutaneous: 4–15 mg q 4–6 hr.
- ii. IV PCA: 0.5–2.5 mg q 6–12 min; 4 hr maximum up to 35 mg. Basal infusion: 0.5–2.0 mg/hr.
- iii. Epidurals: Use only preservative-free morphine preparations. Usual dose range 4–6 mg every 18–24 hr. Important to consider age of patient and surgical incision site. Onset is approximately 30–90 min. Frequently given with 50–100 μg fentanyl, which provides short duration of pain relief until morphine onset.
- iv. Epidural infusion: dose not to exceed 1 mg/hr with or without local anesthetic.
- v. Intrathecal infusion: not to exceed 0.1 mg/hr.
- vi. Intrathecal bolus: 0.2–0.5 mg
- vii. Oral: Elixir, 10–80 mg PO q 4 hr. MS Contin, a controlled-release morphine with a dosage interval of 12 hr: 30 mg q 12 hr is equivalent to 10 mg of elixir q 4 hr.

    d. Pharmacokinetics
- i. IM/SQ: onset, 15–30 min; peak, 45–90 min; duration, 4 hr
- ii. IV: onset, 2–3 min; peak 20 min
- iii. Oral: unreliable absorption—approximately 20% of dose bioavailable
- iv. Epidural: onset, 30–120 min; duration, 18–24 hr
- v. Metabolism: conjugated in kidney and liver (55–80%), demethylation 5%
- vi. Elimination: primarily renal elimination, only 10% biliary excretion, 10% eliminated unchanged; half-life, 1–2 hr

2. **Alfentanil:** Alfentanil is a fentanyl analogue that has one-fifth the potency and one-third the duration of fentanyl.

    a. Side effects
- i. See morphine
- ii. Postoperative confusion, blurred vision, shivering, and hypercapnea have been reported

            iii. may produce bradycardia
      b. Nursing considerations
            i. See morphine
      c. Dosage and administration
            i. PCA/basal infusion: due to short half-life, PCA alfentanil should be combined with basal infusion
           ii. IM/SQ: not routinely used
         iii. Epidural: not routinely used
      d. Pharmacokinetics
            i. Onset after IV injection: 30–45 sec; peak: 1–2 min
           ii. Rapid onset related to low pKa (90% drug is unionized at physiologic pH)
         iii. Volume of distribution is one-fourth that of fentanyl
         iv. Has lower lipid solubility and greater protein binding than fentanyl
          v. Liver metabolism
         vi. Elimination half-life: 1–1.5 hr
        vii. Distribution half-life: 0.4–3.1 min

3. **Fentanyl:** Fentanyl is a synthetic opioid related to the phenylpiperidines. As an analgesic it is estimated to be 75–100 times more potent than morphine.
      a. Side effects
            i. Large IV doses or a bolus dose given rapidly IV may produce marked chest wall rigidity
           ii. See morphine
         iii. May cause bradycardia
      b. Nursing considerations
            i. See morphine
      c. Dosage and administration
            i. IV: Continuous infusion: 1–2 μg/kg/hr.
           ii. PCA: 20–75 μg q 3–10 min, 4 hr limit 0.3 mg. Basal infusion: 10–25 μg/hr
         iii. Epidural: bolus: 25–100 μg in a volume of 10–20 ml. infusion: total dose should not exceed 100 μg/hr, usually combined with bupivacaine with a bupivacaine concentration of 0.02–0.05%
         iv. Intrathecal: 12.5–25 μg bolus
          v. IM/SQ: not routinely used for postoperative analgesia
      d. Pharmacokinetics
            i. IV: onset 30 sec; peak 5–6 min
           ii. IM onset: 7–8 min
         iii. Epidural: onset 5–10 min; duration 1–2 hr

       iv. Intrathecal: onset 1–5 min; duration 1–2 hr
       v. Liver metabolism
      vi. Excreted in bile and urine
     vii. Terminal elimination half-life: 3.0–3.5 hr, reflecting a large volume of distribution

4. **Hydromorphone** (Dilaudid): Hydromorphone is a derivative of morphine which is 8 times more potent, but has a shorter duration of action.
   a. Side effects
      i. See morphine
   b. Nursing considerations
      i. See morphine
   c. Dosage and administration
      i. Oral: 2–4 mg q 4–6 hr
      ii. IM/SQ: 1–2 mg q 4–6 hr
     iii. PCA: 0.1–0.5 mg q 5–15 min, 4 hr dose limit up to 20 mg. Basal infusion: 0.1–0.5 mg/hr
     iv. Epidural: 1 mg q 10–15 hr—Infusions: adults, 50–70 μg/hr; pediatrics, 10 μg/kg/hr. Rectal: 3 mg PR q 6–8 hr.
   d. Pharmacokinetics
      i. Onset (IM) 15–30 min; peaks in 0.5–1 hr; duration is 4–5 hr
      ii. Onset (epidural) 15 min; duration 10–16 hr
     iii. Half-life 2–3 hr
     iv. Metabolized by the liver

5. **Meperidine:** Meperidine is a synthetic opioid agonist, derived from phenylpeperidine. It has approximately one-tenth the potency of morphine.
   a. Side effects
      i. In equianalgesic doses, meperidine produces as much sedation, nausea, respiratory depression, and euphoria as morphine.
      ii. In equianalgesic doses, it may produce less urinary retention and biliary spasm than morphine.
     iii. Contraindicated in patients taking MAO inhibitors
   b. Nursing considerations
      i. See morphine
      ii. With cumulative doses above 1 gr over 24 hr, seizures may occur (2° to the breakdown product normeperidine which has CNS stimulant effects).
   c. Dosage and administration
      i. Oral: 50–200 mg q 3–4 hr

        ii. IM/SQ: 50–150 mg q 3–4 hr

       iii. PCA: 5–20 mg q 6–12 min; 4 hr limit up to 300 mg. Basal infusion: 5–20 mg/hr with PCA.

       iv. Epidural (preservative-free)—bolus, 25–100 mg q 4–6 hr; infusion, at rates up to 15 mg/hr

       v. Intrathecal: 10–20 mg

       vi. Pediatrics: 1.0–1.8 mg/kg IM, SQ or PO every 3–4 hr as needed.

    d. Pharmacokinetics

       i. IM: peak, 30 min to 1 hr; duration, 2–4 hr

       ii. PO: bioavailability 50% peak, 1–2 hr; duration, 4–6 hr

       iii. Epidural: onset, 5–10 min; peak, 15 min; duration, 6–8 hr

       iv. Metabolism: 90% metabolized in the liver by demethylation to normeperidine and hydrolysis to meperidenic acid; <5% excreted unchanged; normeperidine is one-half as active as meperidine, has a CNS stimulant effect and an elimination half-time of 15–40 hr

       v. Elimination half-time: 3–4.5 hr

6. **Methadone:** Methadone is a synthetic opioid agonist with actions quantitatively similar to those of morphine sulfate. When given IV or IM it is equipotent to morphine. It is highly effective when given orally, however only one-half as potent as morphine.

    a. Side effects

       i. See morphine

       ii. Fewer sedative and euphoric effects than morphine

    b. Nursing considerations

       i. Long plasma half-life may result in accumulation with chronic use.

    c. Dosage and administration

       i. IM/SQ: 2.5–10 mg every 3–4 hr

       ii. PO: 5–20 mg every 3–4 hr initially; after 24 hr either decrease dose or increase time interval

       iii. PCA: 0.5–3 mg q 10–20 min; 4 hr limit up to 75 mg. Basal infusion not recommended.

       iv. Epidural: 3–5 mg

       v. Intrathecal: 0.5 mg

    d. Pharmacokinetics

       i. Onset IM 30–60 min; peak 0.5–1 hr

       ii. Highly plasma bound

       iii. Metabolized in liver, then excreted in urine

          iv. Elimination half-time: 15–35 hr

          v. Bioavailability 80%

7. **Oxymorphone (Numorphan):** Oxymorphone is a semisynthetic opioid agonist which possesses many of the attributes of an ideal PCA agent including high analgesic efficacy, rapid onset of effect, and a lower level of sedation. It is 5–10 times more potent than morphine.

    a. Side effects

        i. Contains sodium dithoionite, which may cause allergic reactions

        ii. Causes more nausea and vomiting than morphine

       iii. Risk of physical dependence is great

    b. Nursing considerations

        i. Treatment of nausea and vomiting should be aggressive

    c. Dosage and administration

        i. SQ/IM: 1–1.5 mg q 4–6 hr

        ii. PCA: 0.2–0.3 mg q 6–12 min; 4 hr limit 12 mg. Basal infusion: 0.1–0.2 mg/hr

       iii. Epidural: not used

       iv. Spinal: not used

        v. Rectal: 5–10 mg PR q 4 hr

       vi. Safety and efficacy in children under 12 have not been established.

    d. Pharmacokinetics

        i. IM/SQ: onset 5–10 min; peak 0.5–1 hr; duration 3–6 hr

        ii. *IV*: onset 1/2–2 min

       iii. Half-life; no data available

       iv. Metabolized by the liver

8. **Sufentanil:** Sufentanil is an analogue of fentanyl, with an analgesic potency 5–10 times that of fentanyl. It is more lipid soluble than fentanyl.

    a. Side effects

        i. See morphine

        ii. May cause chest wall rigidity

    b. Nursing considerations

        i. See morphine

    c. Dosage and administration

        i. IM/SQ: not routinely used

        ii. PCA: 2–15 μg every 3–10 min; 4 hr maximum 160 μg. Basal infusion: 1–3 μg/hr

       iii. Epidural: 10–30 μg every 2–4 hr
Infusion: 8–10 μg/hr

        iv. Intrathecal: 1–3 μg

    d. Pharmacokinetics

        i. Greater protein binding than fentanyl (92.5% vs. 84%), therefore, smaller volume of distribution

        ii. Terminal elimination half-life: 2–3 hr

        iii. Metabolized in the liver

B.   OPIOID AGONIST–ANTAGONISTS

   1. **Buprenorphine hydrochloride (Buprenex):** Buprenex is an opioid agonist-antagonist derived from thebaine. Its analgesic potency is approximately 30 times more than morphine. Its antagonism is equipotent to naloxone. It is a partial mu agonist and a kappa antagonist.

    a. Side effects

        i. May precipitate withdrawal in physically dependent individuals

        ii. Sedation occurs in 50% of patients

        iii. Nausea and vomiting in 10–20%

        iv. Respiratory depression *not* reversed with *naloxone*

        v. See morphine

    b. Nursing Considerations

        i. A therapeutic dose of 0.3 mg can decrease respiratory rate similarly to 10 mg of morphine.

        ii. See morphine

        iii. Incompatible with diazepam and lorazepam

    c. Dosage and administration

        i. IM: 0.3–0.6 mg q 6 hr

        ii. PCA: 0.03–0.2 mg q 8–12 min; 4 hr maximum up to 0.8 mg. Basal infusion: 0–0.06 mg/hr

    d. Pharmacokinetics

        i. Onset: IM 15 min; peaks in about 1 hr

        ii. 96% protein bound

        iii. Two-thirds excreted unchanged in bile

        iv. One-third metabolized and then excreted in urine

        v. Half-life is 2–3 hr

   2. **Butorphenol tartrate (Stadol):** Butorphenol is an opioid analgesic with agonist-antagonist activity. The antagonist activity is 1/40 that of naloxone. In potency, 2 mg of butorphenol is equivalent to 10 mg of morphine. It is a mu antagonist and a kappa agonist.

    a. Side effects

        i. Respiratory depression

        ii. Increased PAP, systemic blood pressure, cardiac workload

  b. Nursing considerations
    i. Can cause respiratory depression, headache, and vertigo
    ii. Moderate abuse potential
  c. Dosage and administration
    i. IM: 1–4 mg every 3–4 hr
    ii. IV: 0.5–2 mg every 3–4 hr
    iii. Epidural: 2–6 mg
  d. Pharmacokinetics
    i. Onset: 10 min
    ii. Duration is 3–4 hr
    iii. Metabolized by the liver; excreted primarily in the urine less than 5% is excreted unchanged.

3. **Dezocaine (Dalgan):** Dezocaine (Dalgan) is a synthetic opioid agonist-antagoinst parenteral analgesic of the amino-tetralin series. Its analgesic potency, onset and duration of action in the relief of postoperative pain are comparable to morphine. Peak analgesic effects lags peak serum levels by 20–60 min.

  a. Side Effects
    i. Respiratory depression, which may be reversed with naloxone.
    ii. Contains sodium metabisulfite, that may cause allergic-type reactions.
    iii. May increase ICP in patients with head injuries.
    iv. May cause nausea, vomiting, sedation, dizziness, local irritation at injection sites.
    v. Has not been found to alter cardiac performance.
  b. Nursing Considerations
    i. Produces a similar degree of respiratory depression when compared to morphine.
    ii. May cause delirium in elderly patients.
    iii. Low abuse potential.
  c. Dosage and administration
    i. IM: 10–15 mg every 3–4 hr; dose should be adjusted to the patient's weight, age, severity of pain, physical status, and other medications the patient is receiving; maximum dose in 24 hrs is 120 mg.
    ii. IV: 2.5–10 mg every 2–4 hr
    iii. SQ: not recommended
    iv. Pediatrics and pregnant women: not recommended

      d. Pharmacokinetics
          i. Onset after IM: 10–90 min
          ii. Elimination half-time: 1.7–2.8 hr

4. **Nalbuphine (Nubain):** Nalbuphine is a synthetic opioid agonist-antagonist. It is a potent analgesic, with the same potency as morphine. It depresses respiration as much as equianalgesic doses of morphine, although a ceiling effect occurs such that increases in dosage beyond 30 mg of nalbuphine do not produce further respiratory depression. It is felt to antagonize mu receptors and agonize kappa receptors.

    a. Side Effects
        i. May have abuse potential; abrupt discontinuation of nalbuphine following prolonged use has been followed by symptoms of narcotic withdrawal.
        ii. May precipitate withdrawal in physically dependent individuals
       iii. Contains sodium metabisulfite, which may cause allergic reactions
       iv. See morphine

    b. Nursing Considerations
        i. Very few side effects at ≤10 mg
        ii. See morphine

    c. Dosage and administration
        i. IV, IM, or SQ: 10 mg/70 kg patient q 3–6 hr
        ii. To reverse opioid agonist-induced respiratory depression: nalbuphine should be titrated IV in doses of 2–5 mg every 5 min to desired effect.
       iii. IM/SQ: 10 mg q 3–6 hr
       iv. IV: 10 mg q 3–4 hr
       v. PCA: 1–5 mg q 5–15 min; 4 hr maximum up to 80 mg. Basal infusion: not recommended

    d. Pharmacokinetics
        i. Onset IV: 2–3 min
            Onset IM/SQ: <15 min
        ii. Metabolized in the liver; 7% is excreted unchanged in the urine
       iii. Half-life 5 hr

C. OPIOID ANTAGONIST

1. **Naloxone hydrochloride (Narcan):** Naloxone is an opioid antagonist with a high affinity for the mu receptor. It prevents or reverses the effects of opioids including respiratory depression, sedation, hypotension, as well as pain relief.

    a. Side effects
       i. High doses or abrupt reversal of narcotic depression may induce nausea or vomiting, hypertension, ventricular tachycardia and fibrillation, and pulmonary edema.
      ii. Will produce withdrawal in physically dependent individuals
    b. Nursing considerations
       i. Use with caution in patients with cardiac irritability and narcotic addiction.
      ii. Respiratory depth and rate should be monitored as it is titrated
     iii. Half-life shorter than that of most opioids agonists.
    c. Dosage and administration
       i. To reverse narcotic depression after anesthesia, dose should be titrated to effect in 0.04–0.1 mg IV, SC, or IM boluses.
      ii. Naloxone may be diluted for intravenous infusion in normal saline or dextrose solutions.
     iii. To prophylax against nausea and vomiting and respiratory depression related to neuraxial opioids, infuse at 2–5 μg/kg/hr.
    d. Pharmacokinetics
       i. IV: onset of action within 2 min
      ii. SQ/IM: onset of action slightly more than 2 min
     iii. Duration of action 30–45 min
     iv. Liver metabolism
      v. Elimination half-time: 64 min

III. SEDATIVES/HYPNOTICS
  A. **Diazepam (Valium):** Diazepam, a benzodiazepine, is indicated for the management of anxiety disorders or for short-term relief of symptoms of anxiety, including preoperative anxiety; it may be used to prevent or treat local anesthesia induced seizures; it is a useful adjunct for relief of skeletal muscle spasm caused by reflex spasm to local pathology.
  1. Side effects
    a. Drowsiness, fatigue and ataxia
    b. Venous thrombosis and phlebitis at the IV injection site
    c. Physical dependence can occur
  2. Nursing considerations
    a. Delayed clearance in patients receiving cimetidine

      b. Extreme care must be used in administering intravenous valium because it may cause venous thrombosis, phlebitis, or local irritation

      c. It will potentiate opioid analgesia and side effects

  3. Dosages and administration

      a. Dose should be reduced when a patient is on PCA or receiving epidural/intrathecal opioids.

      b. *Diazepam should not be mixed or diluted with other solutions or drugs in the syringe or infusion flask. It should be administered directly IV.*

      c. PO: 5–25 mg q 6–8 hr

      d. IV: 2.5–10 mg q 4–6 hr

      e. IM: 5–10 mg IM q 3–4 hr. (Erratic absorption after IM administration.)

  4. Pharmacokinetics

      a. Peak effect <1 hr (PO)

      b. Liver metabolism

      c. Elimination half-time: 21–37 hr—prolonged with advanced age and liver disease

B. **Diphenhydramine hydrochloride (Benadryl):** Diphenhydramine hydrochloride is an antihistamine with anticholinergic and sedative effects. It is effective as an antihistamine for treating allergic reactions and in anaphylaxis as an adjunct to epinephrine; it is used to treat motion sickness and other causes of nausea and vomiting.

  1. Side effects

      a. Potentiates alcohol and other CNS depressants

      b. Dizziness, sedation and hypotension

      c. Has an atropine-like action and should, therefore, be used with caution in patients with a histories of bronchial asthma, increased intraocular pressure, hyperthyroidism, cardiovascular disease, hypertension.

      d. MAO inhibitors prolong and intensify the anticholinergic effects of antihistamines

      e. Urinary retention

  2. Nursing considerations

      a. Should be used with caution in patients with narrow-angle glaucoma, and in elderly patients.

  3. Dosage and Administration

      a. Adults: 10–50 mg IV/IM/PO; maximum dose 400 mg/day

      b. Pediatrics: 5 mg/kg/24 hr IV/IM/PO in divided doses; maximum dose 300 mg

4. Pharmacokinetics
   a. Peak plasma concentration: 2–3 hr after PO dose
   b. Duration: 3–6 hr
   c. Elimination half-time: 8 hr
C. **Midazolam (Versed):** Midazolam is a short-acting benzodiazepine. It is indicated for sedation prior to short diagnostic or endoscopic procedures; for induction of general anesthesia; to impair memory of perioperative events; to prevent or treat local anesthetic induced seizures.
   1. Side effects
      a. Respiratory depression
      b. Amnesia
      c. Bigeminy, tachycardia, nodal rhythm
      d. Headache
      e. Nausea/vomiting
      f. Laryngospasm, bronchospasm, dyspnea, wheezing, tachypnea
      g. Confusion, agitation, anxiety, insomnia, muscle tremors, slurred speech
      h. Blurred vision
      i. Hives
   2. Nursing considerations
      a. *Midazolam may cause marked respiratory depression and/or respiratory arrest.*
      b. Potentiated by opioids and barbiturates.
   3. Dosage and administration
      a. IM/IV: Doses may vary from 0.007 to 1 mg/kg. Usually, 10 mg IV will induce general anesthesia in a healthy adult patient.
      b. Midazolam has been used in patient controlled devices.
      c. IV: Dose should be given over at least 2 min.
   4. Pharmacokinetics
      a. Onset IM: 15 min; peak: 30–60 min
      b. Onset IV: 3–5 min
      c. Bioavailability following IM use is >90%
      d. Elimination half-life 1.2–12.3 hr
      e. Less than 0.03% of the dose is excreted intact.
      f. 97% plasma protein bound
IV. NONSTEROIDAL ANTI-INFLAMMATORY DRUGS (NSAIDS): NSAIDs have analgesic and antipyretic activities. The exact mechanism of action is not known, although most agree that the therapeutic activity depends upon inhibition of prostaglandin biosynthesis. All NSAIDs are highly protein bound (>90%). Elimination of NSAIDs depends largely on hepatic biotransformation and excretion is via the

kidneys. Because of potential cross-sensitivity, avoid use in patients in whom aspirin, iodides, or other NSAIDs have induced symptoms of asthma, rhinitis, urticaria, nasal polyps, angioedema, bronchospasm and other allergic symptoms. *Precautions*: (a) NSAIDs can inhibit platelet aggregation—the effect is quantitatively less and of shorter duration than with aspirin. (b) May cause fluid retention and peripheral edema. (c) May cause blurred or impaired vision. (d) May mask signs of infection. (e) Use with caution in patients with abnormal liver function tests. (f) Use cautiously in patients on diuretics. These patients have a greater risk of renal failure secondary to renal blood flow decrease caused by prostaglandin inhibition. (g) May increase the half-life of cimetidine and digoxin.

A. **Ketorolac (Toradol):** Keterolac tromethamine injection is the first commercially available parenteral nonsteroidal antiinflammatory drug (NSAID) marketed for use as a short-term analgesic. Ketorolac is a significant addition to the formulary because it provides potent analgesic effects without opiate-related toxicity.

    1. Nursing considerations
        a. IM injection may result in transient swelling or tenderness (especially with 60 mg loading dose) if the dose is given in the deltoid muscle

    2. Dosage and Administration
        a. Loading doses of 30–60 mg of ketorolac IM should be given followed by half the loading dose of q6 hours IM. IV usage is currently being researched.
        b. Total daily dose of ketorolac should not exceed 120 mg.

    3. Pharmacokinetics
        a. Rapidly absorbed
        b. Onset (IM) 10 minutes
        c. Peak effect (IM): 50 minutes
        d. Half-life 6 hours.
        e. Highly protein bound
        f. Metabolized by the liver; excreted via the kidneys
        g. Side Effects:
            i. GI irritation
            ii. Skin reactions

B. **Ibuprofen** Ibuprofen is indicated for relief of signs and symptoms of rheumatoid arthritis and osteoarthritis; relief of mild to moderate pain; and as an adjuvant to opioid analgesia in moderate to severe postsurgical pain, especially orthopedic surgery.

    1. Nursing considerations
        a. If GI upset occurs, take with meals or milk.

2. Dosage and administration
   a. PO: 300–800 mg tid or qid
   b. Do not exceed 3.2 g/day.
3. Pharmacokinetics
   a. See Ketorolac

V. Other
   A. **Clonidine Hydrochloride** (Catapres) Clonidine is an alpha-adrenergic agonist that has hypotensive effects. The drug lowers coronary vascular resistance, independently of effects on heart rate or myocardial contractility. Bradycardia is rarely severe, and significant arrhythmias are infrequent.

   Clonidine can suppress some components of opioid withdrawal. It is given for 7–10 days (10–25 μg/kg per day) to suppress symptoms, then tapered over 3–4 days. It is most effective in suppressing autonomic symptoms of withdrawal (e.g, nausea, vomiting, diarrhea), than subjective discomfort or craving.

   Clonidine potentiates opioid analgesia and has been used as an adjunct to opioids for pain control.

   TTS - releases a constant rate of drug for 7 days. Therapeutic levels are achieved in 2 to 3 days.

   1. Side Effects
      a. Dizziness, sedation, dry mouth, nausea, indigestion or impotence
      b. CNS
   2. Nursing Considerations
      a. Sudden withdrawal may produce hypertensive crisis
      b. Sympathetic overactivity may occur
      c. May cause dry mouth, sedation, dizziness, fatigue, and headache.
   3. Dosage and Administration
      a. PO: 0.2–0.8 mg daily, administered in 2 or more doses
      b. Transdermal (Catapres TTS): 0.1–0.3 mg/day. Effective for 7 days.
   4. Pharmacokinetics
      a. Rapid and almost complete absorption after oral administration
      b. Peak concentrations in plasma occur 1–3 hours after oral administration.
      c. After transdermal application, peak levels reached in 1–2 days and therapeutic levels persist for 8 hours following removal of TTS.
      d. Plasma half-time: 12.7 ± 7 hours.
      e. Metabolized in the liver; 40% to 60% of the drug excreted unchanged in the urine.

Further information can be found in:

Drug Fact and Comparisons 1989; Facts and Comparisons Div., J.B. Lippincott Co., St. Louis, MO.

The Pharmacological Basis of Therapeutics. Gilman A G, Rall T W, Niew A S, Taylor P. eds., Pergamon Press, NY, 8th Edition, 1990.

Physicians Desk Reference. Schumacher M M ed. Med Economics Co., Inc. NJ, 1991.

Stoelting RK. Pharmacology and Physiology in Anesthetic Practice. J.B. Lippincott Co., Philadelphia, PA 1987.

Appendix 2.2: Products

I. INFUSION DEVICES: Trial evaluations of infusion devices must be arranged through hospital purchasing departments to allow the selection of equipment that will best suit the needs of the acute pain service. Infusion devices can range from a simple nonelectric, disposable device to a highly sophisticated one which allows a variety of delivery modes and dose ranges. Evaluate one type of infusion device at a time, preferably on one nursing unit to allow for better assessment. The following should be considered when choosing equipment:
    A. Pain management modalities with which it will be used
    B. Capability of accommodating proposed modalities
        1. range of doses and basal infusion rates (preprogrammed with minimums or able to program to very low doses)
        2. Program capabilities for mg, μg, ml dosing, or all three
    C. Trial performance
    D. Ease of drug reservoir preparation
        1. Mix or supply opioid as needed or purchase prefilled syringes
        2. Supply 24 hr of patient's opioid requirement or availability of 24-hr pharmacy services
        3. If prefilled syringes are required, the selection of opioids may be limited
    E. User friendliness
    F. Patient convenience
    G. Security of drug
    H. Service and warranty
    I. Reputation of company
    J. Cost
    K. Storage issues
    L. Use as a research tool
        1. Printer availability and/or ability to download to a computer
        2. Programmability for use with nonstandard (investigational) analgesics.

The device chosen must be reliable, easy to use, safe, and provide information on the patient's utilization of the opioid. The company (manufacturer) must stand behind the product with a good service contract, provide reliable, knowledgeable, and available sales personnel to help with inservice programs. The following are various devices available currently

Abbott Laboratories
    1. *LifeCare PCA Plus II—PCA and epidural:* Device has the ability to dose in micrograms or milligrams. PCA, continuous and PCA plus continuous modes.

2. *LifeCare PCA Classic—PCA:* A single-mode PCA infusion device for low-cost PCA procedures
3. *LifeCare Pancretec 5500—PCA and epidural:* Continuous, continuous with bolus, bolus only, intermittent delivery, no captive reservoir, optional lock box.

Bard Medsystems Division

1. *Harvard Bard PCA Pump—PCA and epidural:* PCA, PCA/basal, basal only modes; choice of Bard prefilled or standard Monoject, B-D, 60ml syringes, optional printer.
2. *Bard PCA Pump—PCA and epidural ambulatory:* Program in ml or mg; security code restricts access; programmable in PCA, PCA/basal, or continuous infusion modes; 24 hour history; optional printer.
3. *Bard PCA I—PCA and epidural:* PCA, PCA/basal, basal-only modes; choice of Bard prefilled or standard Monoject, B-D, 60 ml syringes.

Baxter

1. *Stratofuse PCA—PCA and epidural* PCA, continuous, and bolus modes; on-board printer; history; keyed locking system; prefilled syringe.
2. *Basal/Bolus Infusor and PCA Module—PCA and epidural*

Biomedical Products Division Parker Hannifin Corporation

1. *Half Day Infusor and Patient Control Module—PCA:* No programming required; only disposable PCA available; lockout time adjusted by infuser code selection.
2. *Basal/Bolus Infuser and PCA Module—PCA:* No programming required; lockout time adjusted by infuser code selection.

Bionica, Inc.

1. *MDS 110-PCA—PCA only:* Accepts prefilled morphine sulfate syringes; lockable pole mount; security code.

Graseby Medical Ltd.

1. *0125-0701 Graseby Medical PCAs—PCA and epidural:* Includes optional printer, 50/60 ml syringe or 30 ml prefilled syringe.

IVAC Corporation

1. *PCA Infuser, Model 310—PCA and epidural:* Programmable in mg, accepts wide variety of syringes; PCA mode and continuous rate can be used simultaneously or separately.

Medfusion Systems, Inc.

1. *Medfusion—Infumed 300-Ambulatory Infusion Pump—PCA and epidural*
2. *Medfusion 1001-Syringe Infusion Pump—PCA and epidural*
3. *WalkMed 499—PCA and epidural:* Capable of continuous,

continuous intermittent, or continuous/PCA infusions; ideal for chemotherapy, pain management, and antibiotic therapy.

4. *Infu-Med 400 PCA—PCA and epidural:* Ideal for continuous and/or PCA infusions, pain management, and chemotherapy; can be upgraded to include intermittent mode.

5. *Infu-Med 400 I/C—PCA and epidural:* Suitable for intermittent and/or continuous infusions; ideal for antibiotic therapy; can be upgraded to include continuous/PCA mode.

6. *Infu-Med 400—PCA and epidural:* Continuous infusions; ideal for chemotherapy and pain management; upgrade to intermittent and/or PCA; patient lockout kit.

7. *Infu-Med 300—PCA and epidural:* Ideal for ambulatory pain management and chemotherapy; occlusion pressure $10 \pm$ 3psi.

Pharmacia Deltec, Inc.

1. *CADD-PLUS-Ambulatory Infusion Pump—PCA and epidural*

2. *CADD-PCA Ambulatory Infusion Pump, Model 5800—PCA and epidural:* PCA, continuous, and/or clinician bolus; programmable in mg or ml; records doses delivered and attempted.

Strato Medical Corporation

1. *Strato Micropump Ambulatory Medication Infuser 2100—PCA and epidural:* Cassette prevents freeflow, backflow, and air infusion. Patented Flow-Sensor confirms infusion. 100ml and 200ml reservoirs available.

Travenol Laboratories, Inc.

Travenol Infuser with Patient Control Module—PCA only

II. EPIDURAL PRODUCTS

A. Epidural and spinal kits used for postoperative pain management are usually pre-selected, as they are the same as those used in the operating room and in Obstetrics. However, although some institutions use Weiss needles for lumbar epidurals, most institutions will use exclusively Tuohy needles for thoracic epidurals. Thus, in institutions utilizing Weiss needles for lumbar epidural anesthesia, both types of needles must be available for postoperative pain management.

III. SPINAL PRODUCTS

A. Spinal needles: Two basic types of spinal needles are available for use; the standard diamond tipped needle and the blunt tipped needles, "pencil tip" (Whitacre) or "ogval tip" (Sprotte). The major clinical difference between these needles is a lower incidence of post-dural puncture headache (PDPHA) (with the same gauge needle) when using the blunt tipped needles.

B. Spinal catheters: The development of microcatheters has allowed for the use of continuous spinal anesthesia/analgesia without the significant incidence of PDPHA seen historically with 19 gauge catheters. Commercially available microcatheters (27- to 32-gauge) available from Kendall and Preferred Medical Products and may be placed through 22- to 26-gauge diamond tipped or ogval tipped needle.

IV. INTERPLEURAL PRODUCTS: The Arrow Interpleural Kit with Blue FlexTip Interpleural Catheter is the first and only kit designed exclusively for interpleural anesthesia/analgesia. The tip of the Blue FlexTip catheter is more pliant than the remainder of the catheter, and thus minimizes migration and other catheter related complications. The outdwelling catheter segment, also made of polyurethane, is kink resistant and has centimeter markings to aid with catheter placement.

V. PULSE OXIMETERS: Pulse oximeters provide instantaneous measurement of arterial oxygenation by determining the absorpiton characteristics of blood passing between a light source and a photodector. Absorption is measured at two different wave lengths to allow distinguishing between oxyhemoglobin and deoxyhemoglobin. Pulse oximetry is a standard of operating room anesthesiology practice and its use is also often indicated in postoperative pain management. The tremendous market for this product has resulted in a large number of manufacturers producing pulse oximeters. Although not complete, table 2.2 summarizes the features of some of the currently available pulse oximeters.

VI. APNEA MONITORS: The use of apnea monitors is limited, despite their potential usefulness, as all devices have a high likelihood of providing false information. Depending on the type of monitor, it can fail to alarm for apnea or alarm falsely. Apnea monitors are most frequently utilized for monitoring pediatric patients.

TABLE 2.2 Information display, alarms, times, and interference

Brand	Pulsat	Biochem	Bird	Criticare 501	Kontron	Nova-metrix 500	Nelcor 100	Invivo 4500	Data-scope	Ohmeda	Phisio-control	Criticare 502	Nelcor 200	Datex	Radio-meter Oxi
Information display															
Display type	LCD	LED	LCD	LCD	LCD	LCD	LED	LED	LED/LCD	LCD	LED	LCD	LED	CRO	LED
Illuminated	yes	yes	yes	yes	yes	yes	yes	yes	yes	yes	yes	yes	yes	yes	yes
Signal strength	no	no	no	no	yes	yes	yes	yes	yes	yes	yes	yes	yes	no	yes
Pulse waveform	no	no	no	no	no	no	no	no	no	yes	no	yes	no	yes	no
4 meter visibility	Sat	Sat, pulse	Sat	Sat	Sat	Sat, pulse	Sat, pulse	Sat, pulse	Sat, pulse	Sat, pulse	Sat, pulse	Sat, pulse	Sat, pulse	Sat, pulse	Sat, pulse
Variable pitch															
beep	no	no	no	no	no	yes	yes	yes	yes	yes	yes	yes	yes	no	yes
Volume adjust	no	yes	no	no	yes	yes	yes	yes	yes	yes	yes	yes	yes	yes	yes
Beep off	yes	yes	yes	yes	no	yes	yes	yes	yes	yes	yes	yes	yes	yes	yes
Alarm limits displayed	no	no	no	no	yes	yes	no	no	yes	yes	no	no	no	yes	no
Audible alarms off	yes	yes	yes	yes	yes	yes	yes	yes	yes	yes	yes	no	yes	yes	no
Ease of setting alarms	good	good	good	good	good	poor	good	good	good	good	satisfactory	satisfactory	good	good	good
What alarms settable	Sat	Sat, pulse	Sat	Sat	Sat, pulse	Sat, pulse	Sat, pulse	Sat, pulse	Sat, pulse	Sat, pulse	Sat, pulse	Sat, pulse	Sat, pulse	Sat, pulse	Sat, pulse
Alarm silence (min)	3	2	3	3	reset/off	2	1–2	1	1	0.5	1	2	1–2	2	3
Alarm limits															
Sat low	80–95	60–90	80–95	80–95	50–95	0–95	50–100	50–100	70–95	50–100	50–100	1–99	50–100	40–99	21–100
High	no	95–97	80–95	no	70–100	5–100	85–100	70–100	80–100	70–100	50–100	86–100	52–100	76–100	85–100
Heart rate low	no	30–100	no	no	30–150	30–245	35–206	20–200	30–100	40–200	20–150	20–79	35–55	30–250	1–120
High	no	125–275	no	no	50–250	35–250	55–250	70–250	100–250	70–250	80–240	80–250	55–250	30–250	70–250
Times/interference															
Attach-first reading	9	15	5–7	10	7	13	5–8	6	6	15	4–10	5	6	5	9
Removal- blank screen	3	20	2	2–20	2	1	9	6	8	2	1	2	15–20	4	3
Removal-alarm	3	19	2	2–20	2	1	9	3	17	2	1	2	15–20	24	2
Diathermy effect	good	satisfactory	good	good	satisfactory	good	good	good	good	satisfactory	good	good	good	good	satisfactory
Light effect	good	good	good	good	good	poor	satisfactory	poor	good	good	good	good	satisfactory	satisfactory	good

Reproduced with permission from Morris RW, Nairn M, Torda TA. A comparison of fifteen pulse oximeters. Part I: A clinical comparison; Part II: A test of performance under conditions of poor perfusion. *Anaesth Intens Care* 1989;17:62–82.

Appendix 2.3: Company Addresses and Products

Company addresses	Products
Abbott Laboratories P.O. Box 8500 S-6665 Philadelphia, PA 19178	Infusion devices, epidural/spinal catheter and kits
Arrow International, Inc. Hill and George Avenues Reading, PA 19610	Epidural/spinal catheters, interpleural catheters and kits
Bard MedSystems Division 87 Concord Street North Reading, MA 01864	Infusion devices
Baxter Healthcare Corporation Pharmacy Division 1425 Lake Cook Road Deerfield, IL 60015	Infusion devices
Baxter/Fenwall Laboratory P.O. Box 3836 Boston, MA 02241	Infusion devices, epidural/spinal catheters and kits
Becton Dickenson Respiratory Systems P.O. Box 98804 Chicago, IL 60693	Epidural/spinal catheters and kits, infusion devices
Biomedical Products Parker Hannifin Corporation 17352 Von Karman Avenue Irvine, CA 92741	Epidural catheters
Bionica, Inc. 28636 Jaeger Drive Laguna Niguel, CA 92677	PCA devices
Burron Medical, Inc. P.O. Box 8500 S-2386 Philadelphia, PA 19178	Epidural/spinal catheters and kits
Concord/Protex P.O. Box 8500 (S-5155) Philadelphia, PA 19178	Portex/RSP, epidural/spinal catheters and kits

Davol, Inc.
P.O. Box 75677
Charlotte, NC 28275

Epidural/spinal catheters and kits,
    infusion devices

Edentec
10252 Valley View Road
Eden Prairie, MN 55344

Apnea monitors

Graseby Medical Ltd.
124 Maryland Route #3, Suite 9
Millersville, MD 21108

Apnea monitors, infusion devices

Kendall Company
P.O. Box 8765
New York, NY 10049

Epidural/spinal catheters and kits,
    microcatheters

Medfusion Systems, Inc.
3450 River Green Court
Duluth, GA 30136

Infusion devices

Nellcor, Inc.
25495 Whitesall Street
Hayward, CA 94545

Pulse oximeter

Nonin Medical, Inc.
13030 Highway 55
Plymouth, MN 55441

Pulse oximeter

Novametrix Medical Systems
Barnes Industrial Park
Wallingford, CT 06492

Pulse oximeter

PMT Corporation
P.O. Box 75867
Charlotte, NC 28275

Epidural/spinal catheters and kits,
    spinal microcatheters

Pharmacia Deltec, Inc.
1265 Grey Fox Road
St. Paul, MN 55112

Infusion devices

Sheridan Catheter Corp.
Rt. 40
Argyle, NY 12809

Epidural/spinal catheters and kits

IMD International Medical & Dental, Inc. 3380 Agar Place Bronx, NY 10465	Sprotte spinal needles
Strato Medical Corporation 123 Brimbul Avenue Beverly, MA 01915	Infusion devices
Sherwood Medical P.O. Box 75867 Charlotte, NC 28275	Spinal needles and spinal trays
Travenol Laboratories, Inc. Deerfield, IL 60015	Infusion devices, epidural/spinal kits
Vygon Corp. 1 Madison Street East Rutherford, NJ 07073	Epidural/spinal catheters, epidural/spinal needles

Subject Index